THE CAUSE OF THYROID DISEASE

SURESH KORADA

McCLELLAND
www.mcclelland.in

First published: 2022

ISBN 978-93-5759-917-7

Printed and bound at Parksons Graphics Pvt. Ltd.,

Caution: The purpose of the book is to provide information and analysis. It is not intended to be medical advice. You should consult your physician for medical advice. Every patient is unique and his or her circumstances are unique. Only your physician will be able to advice the best approach for your specific needs and circumstances.

Front cover: Limestone quarry at Akselberget, Brønnøy, Norway
Credit: Thomas Bjørkan

Back cover: Limestone rocks and slate rock
Credit: Adobe stock

Contents

Acknowledgments

Dolores Campanario, World Health Organization (WHO) Permissions Department, for permission to adapt content from the monograph series on endemic goiter, published by WHO in 1960. This specific content is from the research work of Kelly F.C. and Snedden W.W., Langer P., and Clements F.W.

Anju Sharma, Editor-in-Chief, *Indian Journal of Medical Research*, and Albina Nair, scientist, *Indian Journal of Medical Research*, for helping me retrieve the research work of Scott H., Gupta S.P., et al. from 1931 and 1934.

EUMETSAT, the European operational satellite agency, for permission to use topography maps of various countries.

Venkataraman Anantharaman, for copyediting.

Laura Brecher, for internal book design and illustrations.

Introduction

Thyroid disease has become rampant in recent times. In the United States, for which data is available, about 20 million people, or roughly 6% of the population, take synthetic thyroid hormone medication for thyroid disease.[1] Since thyroid disease primarily affects women, we may estimate that over 12% women in the United States take synthetic thyroid medication.

In this book, we will focus on *the cause* of thyroid disease. And among various thyroid diseases, we will focus on hypothyroidism. Hypothyroidism is a disease in which a decreased quantity of thyroid hormone is produced by the thyroid gland.

A brief explanation is required for the two new words that we just introduced—gland and hormone. A gland is an organ that produces a juice-like substance. The juice-like substance is called hormone. The salivary glands and sweat glands are examples of glands that we can normally see and feel. There are other glands that we cannot feel, as they are located deep inside our body. The thyroid gland is an example of such an internal gland located at the base of the front neck. The thyroid gland produces thyroid hormones. These hormones are released into the blood stream. Glands that release their hormones into the blood are called endocrine glands. Hence, the thyroid gland is an endocrine gland.

The cause of thyroid disease is commonly attributed to iodine deficiency. But if iodine deficiency was the cause of thyroid disease, then most of the world should have been free of thyroid disease, as many countries across the world have been adding iodine to salt for the last hundred years. In the United States, for example, there is an excess consumption of iodine in the form of various iodine-rich foods such as milk and

1 Wallach O. Ranked: The Most Prescribed Drugs in the US (Based on data from U.S. Agency for Healthcare Research and Quality, released in 2021 for the 2019 calendar year). visualcapitalist.com. https://www.visualcapitalist.com/ranked-the-most-prescribed-drugs-in-the-u-s/ Accessed April 29, 2022.

fast food. Yet, thyroid disease is rampant in the United States. Make no mistake, iodine is important for thyroid health. Iodine is present both in the thyroid gland and in thyroid hormones in significant amounts. But deficiency of iodine is not the cause of thyroid disease.

More recently, the cause of thyroid disease has been attributed to autoimmunity—a condition in which the immune system attacks the body's own organs. Per autoimmunity theory, the immune system attacks the thyroid gland, resulting in thyroid disease. However, autoimmune condition may be an effect of thyroid disease rather than the cause. Autoimmunity may be a *symptom* of the disease, rather than the cause.

Whatever the cause of thyroid disease be, it should explain the large number of symptoms associated with the disease. *The cause* discussed in this book will account for all the symptoms, while iodine deficiency and autoimmunity fail to explain even a handful of the symptoms observed in thyroid disease. We will see during the course of this book that the cause of thyroid disease is not due to a *deficiency*, but to *an excess* of something. I hope the findings in this book will fundamentally change our understanding of thyroid disease.

Chapter 1

History of Thyroid Disease

Thyroid disease is as old as the mountains.

Two thousand years ago, all the major civilizations of the past—China, India, and Europe—made references to thyroid disease.[1] Such a long historical record shows that thyroid disease is a very old disease. Whatever the cause of thyroid disease be, the cause existed two thousand years ago, and it still exists today. The historical record also shows that thyroid disease and its cause existed in all major countries of the world, it was not restricted to any particular country or region.

Three thousand years ago

It is difficult to imagine life three thousand years ago. Life, food, clothes, and homes may have been very primitive. Yet, from such early times, we have a written record of thyroid disease.

The earliest known written record of thyroid disease is from China. This record is from the Shang Dynasty, which ruled China 3,600 years ago, from 1600 BC to 1046 BC. Much of the written history of the Shang Dynasty is deciphered from the inscriptions on oracle bones (animal bones and tortoise shells). About 4,500 different words have been discovered from these bones. One of the words was *Ying*, which was interpreted as a bump on the neck.[2] The bump on the neck was *goiter*, a severe form of thyroid disease. We will discuss about goiter in detail in the next chapter.

About the same time, in India too, there has been a reference to goiter. In Atharva Veda, an ancient Indian text, which dates to about 3,000 years ago (1000 BC), incantations for goiter disease have been found.[1(p10)] The Atharva Veda is a repository of procedures for everyday life. It is a collection of 730 hymns containing about 6,000 verses, divided into 20 books.[3]

Two thousand years ago

Let us travel a thousand years in time to see if our ancestors had made any progress in their understanding of thyroid disease. About the 4th century BC, i.e., about 2,400 years ago, we find the first reference to *the cause* of thyroid disease. In the book *The Classic of Mountains and Seas* (Chinese, *Shan Hai Jing*), there is mention of goiter disease. The book attributes *the cause* of goiter to *poor quality of water.*[1(p9)]

In the 4th century BC, we also find the first reference to goiter in Europe. The reference is found in *Air, Water, and Places*, a treatise by Hippocrates, a renowned physician of ancient Greece. This treatise too mentions *drinking water* as *the cause* of goiter.[1(p11)]

In the 1st century BC, i.e., 2,100 years ago, Vitruvius, a famous Roman architect and civil engineer, wrote, "The Aequi in Italy and Medulli in the Alps have *a kind of water,* from drinking which they get a kind of swelling."[1(p10,11)] The Alps is the tallest mountain range in Europe.

In the 1st century AD, i.e., 1,900 years ago, Pliny, an author, natural philosopher, and army and naval commander of early Roman Empire, wrote on the subject of goiter: "Swelling of neck occurs only in men and in swine, caused mostly *by water they drink.*"[1(p13)] This record also shows that water is the cause of thyroid disease and that animals too suffered from thyroid disease.

In the 2nd century AD, i.e., 1,800 years ago, Ulpianus, a Roman jurist and one of the greatest legal authorities of his time, wrote, "The inhabitants of the Alps suffer from a big neck, *caused by the quality of water they drink.*"[1(p11)] Again, in the 2nd century AD, there is a reference to the location where the disease occurred. In China, in the Han Dynasty (206 BC to AD 220) and in the Wei Dynasty (AD 200–264), drinking water and certain conditions of life in the *mountainous regions* were referred to as the causes of thyroid disease.

Seven hundred years ago

About the year 1300, Guido Lanfranchi, who is regarded as the founder of surgery in France, considered *hard water*, especially that found in the Alps, to be *the cause* of goiter.[1(p13)] This was, perhaps, one of the first references to *hard water* as the cause of thyroid disease.

Five hundred years ago

Paracelsus (1493–1541) described goiter and attributed the disease to a deficiency of minerals in water.[1(p13)] This was probably the first time someone said that a *deficiency of minerals* in water was the cause of thyroid disease.

A description of the *most* severe form of thyroid disease—cretinism—was made by Felix Platter (1536–1614) of Basle, Switzerland.[1(p13)] We will discuss cretinism in detail in the next chapter. Cretinism had certainly existed before five hundred years; it was, however, described for the first time about five hundred years ago.

In 1656, Thomas Wharton, a London anatomist, introduced the term *thyroid*. It was derived from the Greek word *thyreos*, meaning a shield, based on the thyroid gland's shield-like appearance wrapped in the front of the trachea/throat.[4]

Two hundred years ago

In 1873, the first clear description of the milder form of thyroid disease, myxedema, was given by William Gull (1816–1890), as "a cretinoid state supervening in the adult life of a woman." He was the first one to use the word *hypothyroidism*, which we now commonly use to refer to the low-thyroid-hormone disease.

Local people

In all the above discussion, we have seen the progress of thyroid disease through the eyes of the great men of the past. But ordinary people are also a good source to know the cause of a local disease. They live through generations in the same location. They would know better about local diseases than observers or researchers who come there for a short while to study a disease. What did local people believe *caused* thyroid disease? About the year 1835, in India, per the research of the British medical doctor John McClelland, the local people (natives) attributed the prevalence of goiter to *the impurity of particular waters.*[5] Around 1855, in Europe, the popular belief among common people in many places *laid the blame on the waters.*[6(p5)] Khol, a German traveler, mentioned that in Styria, Austria, the popular explanation of goiter and cretinism *tended to throw the blame upon the water*, for the peasantry shunned drinking from many springs and traveled far to find others; they said that out of the condemned springs arose *stupidity.*[6(p31)] Thus, local people identified *drinking water* as the *cause* of thyroid disease.

In summary, from the brief historical note, we may say that thyroid disease is a very old disease, and *the cause* of thyroid disease lies in drinking water.

References

1. Langer P. History of goitre. In: *Endemic Goitre.* Monograph Series No. 44. Geneva: World Health Organization; 1960:9-25
2. Baoshan Z, Binbin W, Finkelman RB. Medical geology in China: Then and now. In: Selinus O, Finkelman R, Centeno J, eds. *Medical Geology. A Regional Synthesis.* Springer; 2010:305
3. Bloomfield M. *The Atharvaveda.* Verlag von Karl J Trübner; 1899:1-2
4. Ellis H. The early days of thyroidectomy. *J Perioper Pract.* 2011;21(6):215-216. doi: 10.1177/175045891102100606.

5. McClelland J. An inquiry into the nature and causes of goitre. In: *Some Inquiries in The Province of Kemaon, Relative to Geology, and Other Branches of Natural Science.* Calcutta: Thacker & Co. and Cantor & Co.; 1835:268-269

6. Blackie GS. *Cretins and Cretinism, A Prize Thesis of the University of Edinburgh*. Edinburgh: Maclachlan & Stewart, and London: Simpkin, Marshall & Co.; 1855

Chapter 2

Thyroid Diseases

i. Goiter

Goiter is a severe form of thyroid disease.

People in the past did not have the diagnostic tests we have today. Then, how did people know that they had thyroid disease? Well, the disease was visible to the naked eye; there was a swelling around the neck. This swelling of neck is a disease called *goiter*. As science progressed, we got to know that the swelling of the neck was actually a swelling of the thyroid gland. The thyroid gland is located just below the front neck. If it was just a swelling of neck or thyroid gland, we would not have worried so much. But the swelling was usually accompanied by other symptoms that were problematic.

In goiter, the thyroid gland functions below its normal potential. As a result, the body functions below its normal potential. Men and women with goitres were sluggish and easily tired. They were characterized by a want of enterprise and bodily vigor in comparison with their immediate neighbors, who did not have goiter.[1(p367)] In goiter, both the body and the mind become sluggish. Further, goiter is associated with deficient speech and hearing, rheumatic joint pains, puffy face, and bloated body.

These symptoms are not different from what we call hypothyroidism today. Hypothyroidism is subnormal function of the thyroid gland, resulting from a decreased quantity of thyroid hormone produced by the thyroid gland. The difference between goiter and hypothyroidism is the degree of severity of symptoms and the absence of swelling of neck in hypothyroidism. Figures 2.1 to 2.4 show people with goiter.

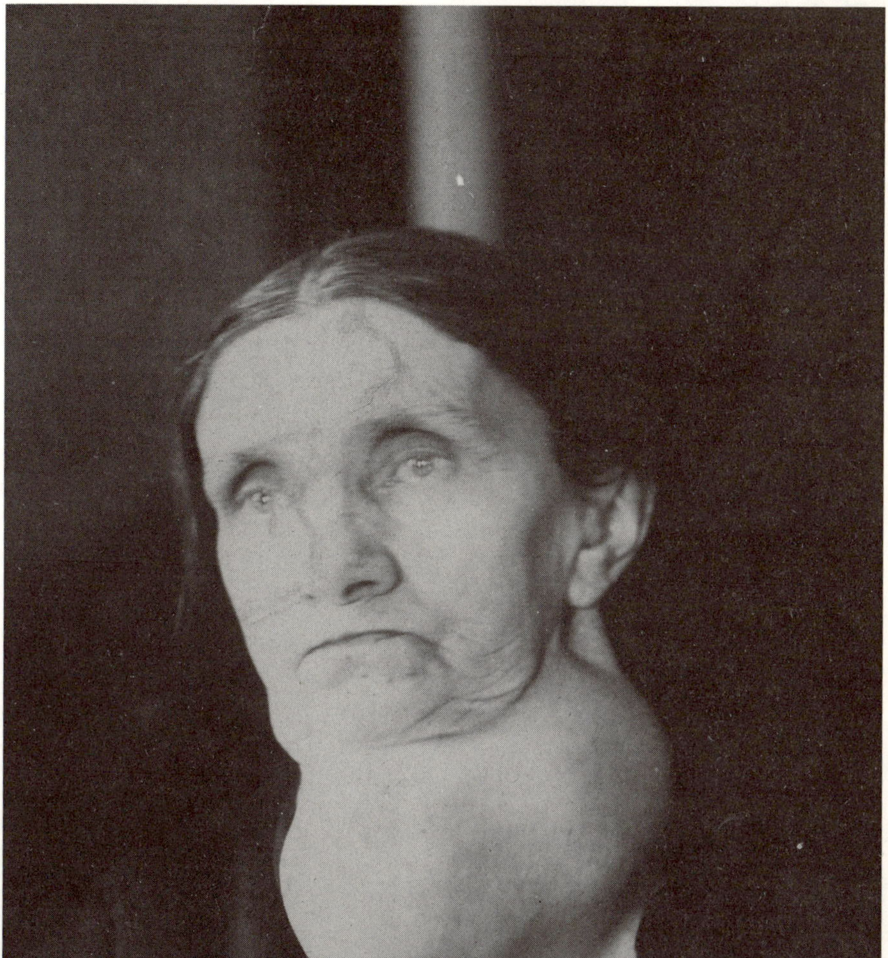

Figure 2.1 Woman aged 64 years, with goiter of long standing.[2]
St Bartholomew's Hospital Archives and Museum, London.
Credit: Wellcome collection

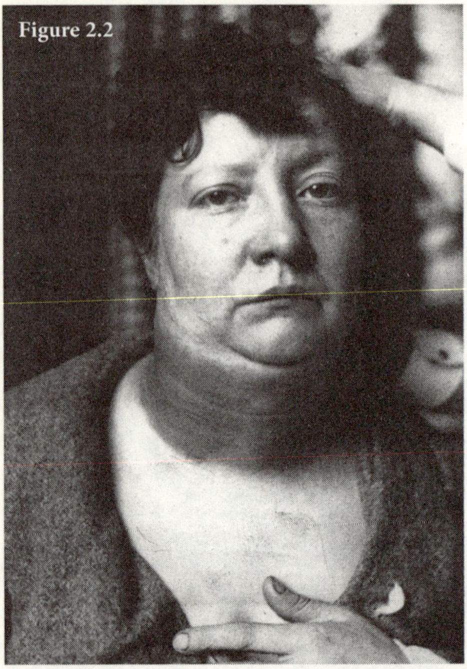

Figure 2.2
Woman with goiter.[3]

Figure 2.3
Boy with goiter.[4]

Figure 2.4
Girl with large goiter.[5]

Images credit:
St Bartholomew's Hospital
Archives and Museum, London
Wellcome collection

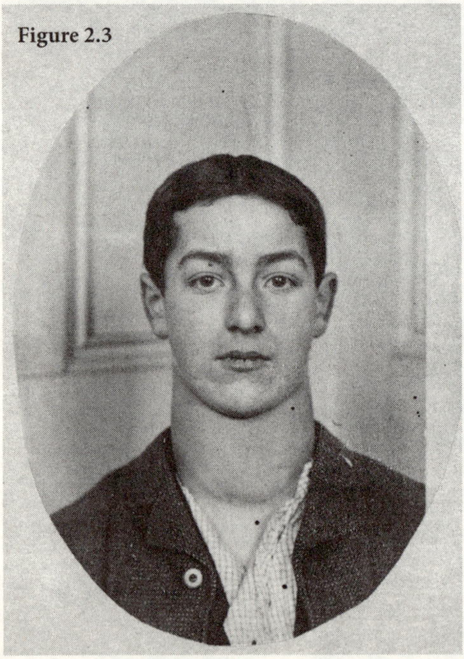

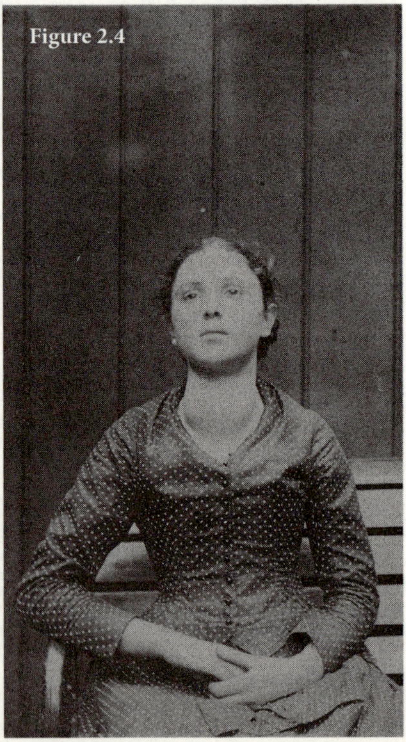

ii. Cretinism

The most severe form of thyroid disease is cretinism. A person suffering from cretinism is called a cretin. In cretinism, no organ in the body functions normally. It is surprising that such a massive disruption is brought about by the malfunctioning of a small gland, the thyroid gland.

Felix Platter coined the term *cretin* to describe the particular kind of people he noticed in sufficient numbers in the valleys of the Alps.[6(p246)] His description covered the salient features of cretinism: disproportionate body, large head, short limbs, immense tongue, deaf-mutism, and mental retardation. He recognized that not all cretins had goiter. In 1954, it was noted in Cameroon, Africa, that only 23% of cretins had goiter.[7(p76)] This shows that thyroid gland enlargement does not always occur in thyroid disease.

In McClelland's research in India, he found that when goiter prevailed in more than 50% of a population, there were about 30% cretins in that population. And where goiter prevalence was less than 9%, there were no cretins in that population.[1(p371)]

The symptoms of cretinism as described by various observers over the past three hundred years are listed below. You may take a note of these symptoms because we find similar symptoms in hypothyroidism, which is the common form of thyroid disease today, only that the severity of symptoms is much less in hypothyroidism than in cretinism.

The symptoms of cretinism may be broadly categorized as those affecting the body and the brain.[8]

Body

The visible human body is primarily made of bones, muscles, and skin. Bones are the scaffolding that hold the human body in an erect position. Cretinism affects this very structure. Most bones are deformed in a cretin. The head is of unusual size. It is too big in proportion to the rest of the body. The top of the skull is flattened. The face bones are large and very prominent. The extreme ends of long bones in the legs and hands are broad and large relative to the rest of the long bone. There is swelling at the joints. The spinal cord is usually curved. The chest bones are narrow and crooked. The fingers are short. The knees are bent forward and inward. The feet are flat. As a result, the walk of a cretin is difficult, tottering, and uncertain. There is no symmetry in the structure of the whole body. In hypothyroidism, rheumatic bone/joint pains are a common symptom.

The skin acts as the outer shield to the human body. In cretins, the skin of the whole body is thick, flabby, and sagging. The cretin always feels cold and tends to instinctively seek the sun and bask in its rays. This excess feeling of chill is a symptom even in hypothyroidism.

Muscles hold the skin to the bones. In a cretin, all muscles are weakened.

In addition to the *structure* of the body, the *functioning* of the body is disrupted in cretinism. A cretin lacks energy. He's lazy and indolent. Lack of energy and tiredness is a common symptom even in hypothyroidism.

Brain

In a cretin, the brain is equally or even more adversely afflicted than the body.

The sensory organs provide inputs to the brain for its decision-making, in turn, the sensory organs get their instructions from the brain. *Dullness of the senses and nonfunctional senses* is the common theme in a cretin. A cretin is usually deaf and mute, or there is imperfection in speech. In a few, there is stuttering and stammering. Parents affected with stammering, a very common disorder in the Valais, Switzerland, often had a cretin offspring.

In the absence of proper sensory inputs, the brain is unable to perform its normal functions. In cretins, there is no comprehension ability. Cretins do not properly comprehend what they see or hear. The cretins show no power of reasoning or any instinctive reasoning ability. Love, affection, and gratitude are unknown sentiments to a cretin; instead, cretins are cowardly, deceitful, resort to cheating and commit petty offenses.

Symptoms of cretinism as described by early observers of the disease

John McClelland

About 1835, a British medical doctor, John McClelland, observed in Kumaon at the foothills of Himalayas in northern India the following symptoms in cretins. "The cretins in Kumaon are characterized by general deformity of the body. In cretins, the head is often of enormous size, the limbs are short and crooked, the joints are large, and the spine is distorted. There is monstrous development of certain organs, while natural growth of others is distorted. The abdomen is swollen. The thyroid gland in cretins is mostly enlarged, but not always. The mental faculties are feeble and sometimes idiotic. The look on the face of cretins is vacant and stupid."[1(p368–372)]

Berchtold Beaupré

In 1842, a description of cretinism was given by Berchtold Beaupré of Fribourg, Switzerland, in his *Essay on Cretins* (French: *Dissertation sur les Cretins*). Beaupré noted that "cretins bear the human form in its lowest expression." He described the disease as it occurred in the lower parts of Fribourg, where it was endemic. The following is the summary of his observations.[9(p15–16)]

Bones

Head is of unusual size and form; and drops listlessly onto the breast. Nose is flat. Chest is narrow. Back is curved. Arms and legs are short, misshapen, lean, stiff, without power, and without vitality. Knees are thick and inclined inward. Feet are flat.

Body

Figure is squat and bloated. Skin is dirty and flabby, covered with tetters (reddish eruptions such as in eczema). Eyelids are thick and projecting. Teeth are about to decay. Tongue is thick and hangs down. Mouth is always open and full of saliva. Lips are moist and livid. Breath is asthmatic. Belly resembles a bag and seems so loose that it cannot retain the intestines in the cavity.

Brain and senses

Eyes are hollow and heavy. The look is stupid. Hearing is limited. A cretin utters only a hoarse, wild inaccurate sound.

Behavior

A cretin shows greediness. One passion alone he seems to have and that is the sexual instinct, in its rudest brutality.

François-Emmanuel Fodéré

In 1792, Fodéré, a French doctor, in his *Essay on Goiter and Cretinism* (French: *Traité du Goitre et du Crétinisme*), made the following observations on symptoms, in addition to those made by the earlier observers.[5(p16–18)] Fodéré worked in Saint-Jean-de-Maurienne, a French commune in the department of the Savoie in Auvergne-Rhône-Alpes of France, a location surrounded by high mountains on all sides.

Body

Head is large and out of proportion to the rest of the body; it is flattened at the summit and the temples. Chest is flat. Hands are larger than natural.

There is an incipient goiter in the neck in the first years. There is a puffed, swollen countenance of face and body. Puberty comes very slowly, with enormous genitals. Life span is usually short; a few, however, live long lives.

Brain and senses

Eyes are small, sometimes deeply sunk, at other times prominent. A cretin is deaf and mute. The most revolting odors scarcely affect a cretin.

Behavior

A cretin shows repetitive behavior; he can take no other road than that with which he is familiar. We know that repetitive behavior is a common symptom in autism. A cretin is in a habitual state of stupor and sloth.

Cretins are obstinate; they have a mutinous temper. They show no gratitude for the good offices rendered to them and scarcely show any sensibility at the sight of their relations.

Figures 2.5 to 2.8 show people with cretinism.

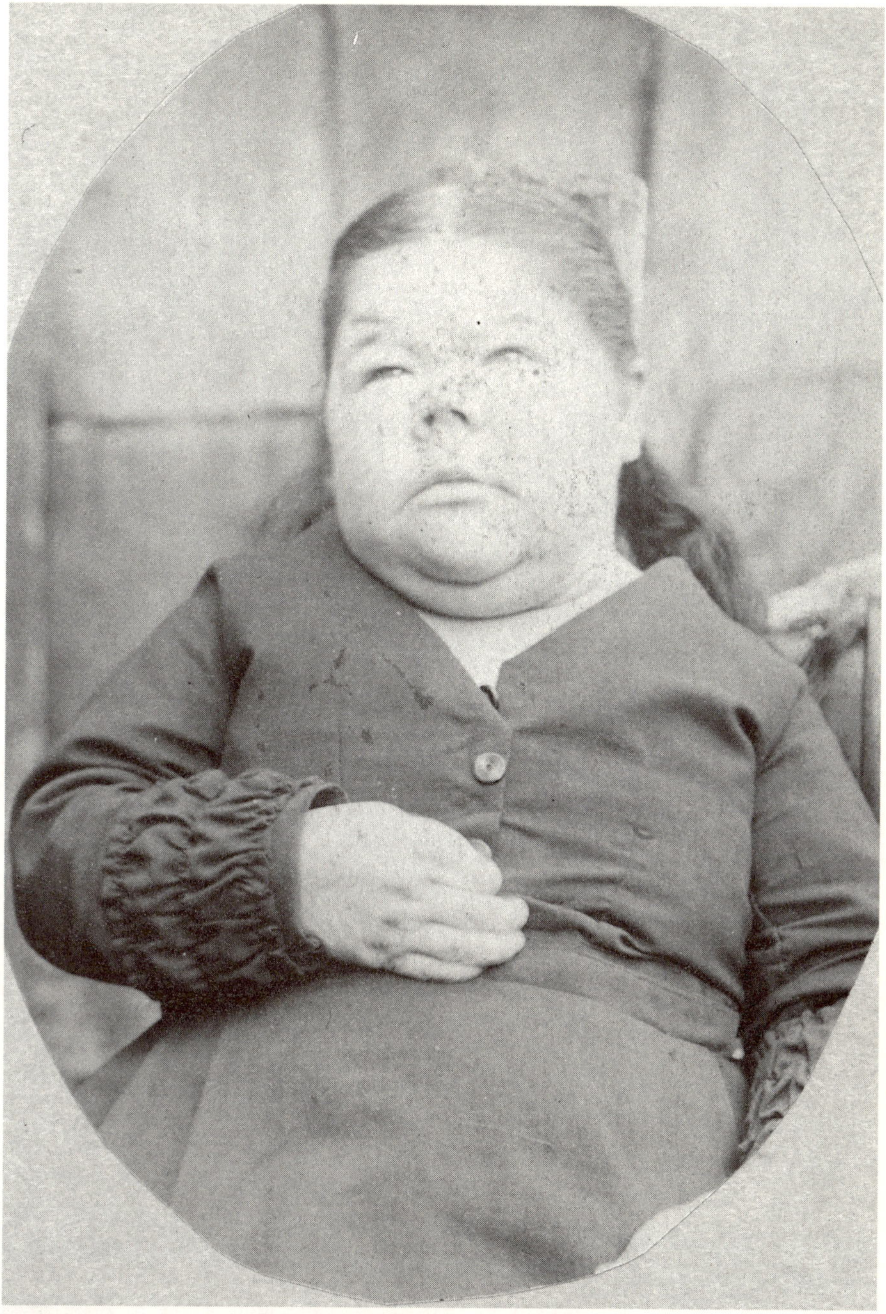

Figure 2.5 Cretin, female, aged 25, a native of Steeple Aston, Wiltshire, England.[10]
St Bartholomew's Hospital Archives and Museum, London.
Credit: Wellcome collection

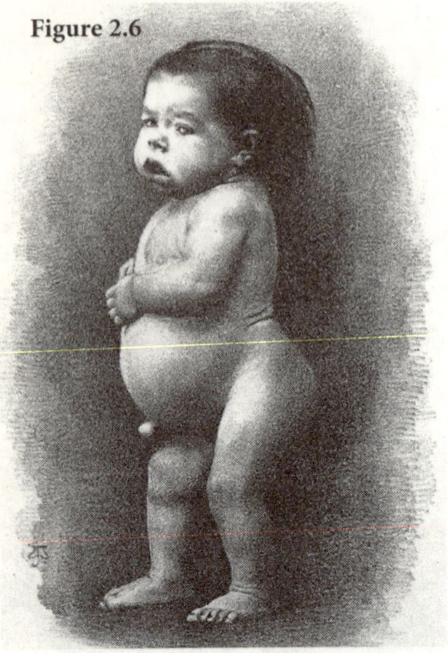

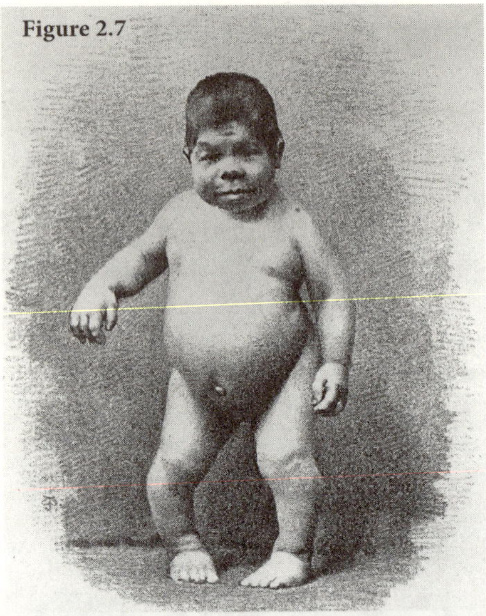

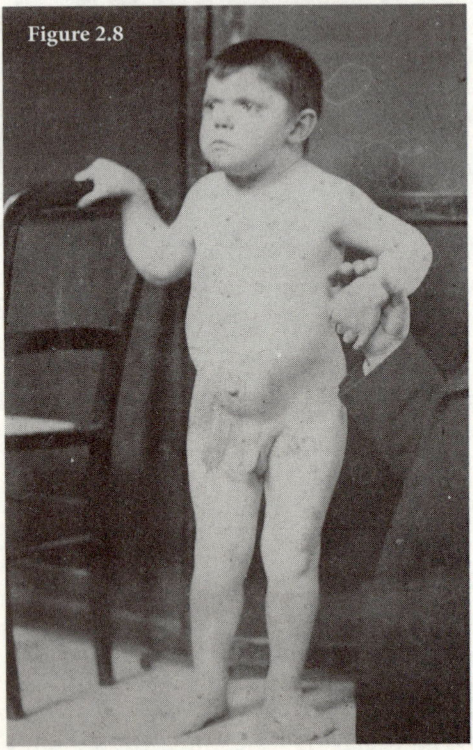

Figure 2.6 Cretin, girl, photo dated 1892–1896.[11]

Atlas of clinical medicine. By Sir Byrom Bramwell.
Credit: Wellcome collection.

Figure 2.7 Cretin, boy, photo dated 1892–1896.[12]

Atlas of clinical medicine.
By Sir Byrom Bramwell.
Credit: Wellcome collection.

Figure 2.8 Cretin, believed to be aged 16 years.[13]

St Bartholomew's
Hospital Archives and Museum, London.
Credit: Wellcome collection

Johann Georg Kohl

In 1842, Johann Georg Kohl, a German traveler, in his *Hundred Days of Travel* (German: *Hundred Tage auf Reisen*), described cretins in Styria, Austria. The following is the summary of his observations.[5(p14–15)]

Body

Stature is short, neck is with goiter, legs are bent, the walk is clumsy and slow, appetite is most voracious, and sexual propensities are manifested in the most brutal and disgusting way.

Senses

Eyes are dull and listless. Hearing is seldom acute.

Brain

Memory and desire for knowledge are vanished. A cretin is without a feeling, without a thought, and is malicious, revengeful, and cruel.

Another German traveler, Weber, in his great work on Germany, alluded to the subject of cretinism. Weber, a more practical traveler, almost reiterated the above statements, and ended by saying that cretins *are midway between man and beasts.*[5(p15)] It is surprising that malfunctioning of a simple gland such as the thyroid gland can make someone seem midway between man and beast.

iii. Hypothyroidism

Hypo means *low*. Hypothyroidism is low thyroid gland function. When one suffers from hypothyroidism, the thyroid gland produces low quantity of thyroid hormone. In hypothyroidism, the severe symptoms of goiter or cretinism may not be present, but many symptoms are common between goiter and cretinism and hypothyroidism.

The following are the common symptoms of hypothyroidism:

Fatigue: Fatigue is the defining symptom of hypothyroidism. A person suffering from hypothyroidism feels less energy and extreme tiredness throughout the day. The person has to drag herself/himself to initiate or complete tasks at work or home.

Brain Fog: The brain of a person suffering from hypothyroidism is foggy and sluggish. The person is unable to think clearly and is unable to take decisions; hence, decision-making is hampered. Thus, in hypothyroidism, it is not just the body that is fatigued; even the mind is fatigued.

Constipation: Constipation is another defining symptom of hypothyroidism.

Puffy body: The entire body is bloated, as if water has accumulated. The face is puffy, and the skin is thick and flabby. A puffy face is the common visible symptom of hypothyroidism.

Low body temperature: Another defining symptom of hypothyroidism is the excessive feeling of cold, even when others around are not experiencing cold.

Joint pain: In hypothyroidism, there is pain in the joints, especially in knee, ankle, elbow, shoulder, and wrist joints. The joint pain is similar to rheumatic joint pain, originating both in the bone and muscle.

Muscle spasms: In hypothyroidism, there are frequent instances of numbness, muscle spasms and cramps.

Weight gain: A person suffering from hypothyroidism puts on weight and is unable to lose it.

Hypothyroidism affects more women than men. Women, in general, are conscious of their skin, hair, and nails and it in these areas hypothyroidism's visible affects are seen.

Skin: The skin is dry and rough. White flakes form on the rough dry skin. It loses its shine/radiance.

Hair: The hair becomes weak and falls out.

Nails: The nails are thin and brittle, and often show cracks.

Sexual dysfunction: In a person suffering from hypothyroidism, there is often sexual dysfunction and infertility.

Senses: In a person suffering from hypothyroidism, the sharpness of senses, especially hearing, sight, and speech, are diminished.

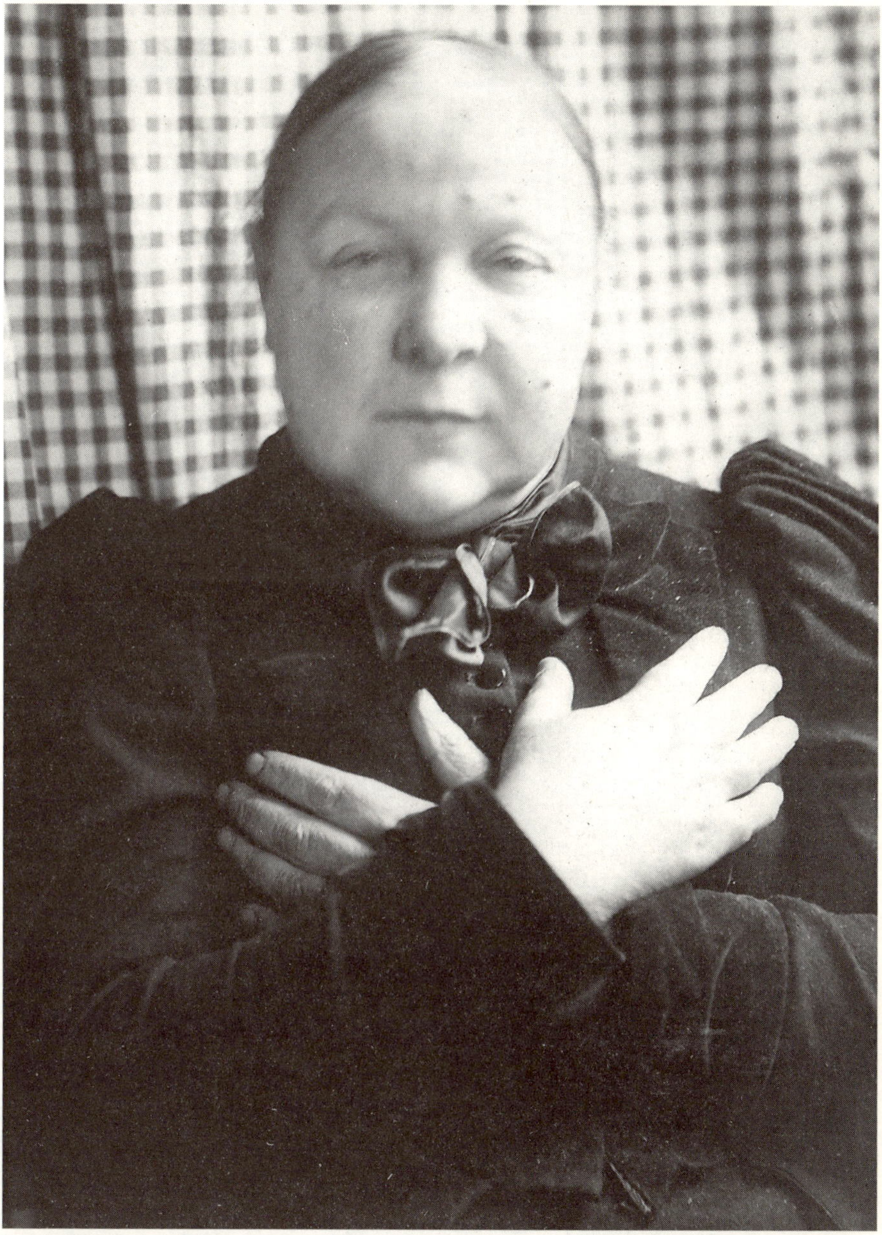

Figure 2.9 The face and hands of a woman, aged 47, suffering from well-marked myxoedema (hypothyroidism). Photograph taken by James Hussey, physician, whilst a student at St Bartholomew's Hospital Medical School.[15]
St Bartholomew's Hospital Archives and Museum, London.
Credit: Wellcome collection

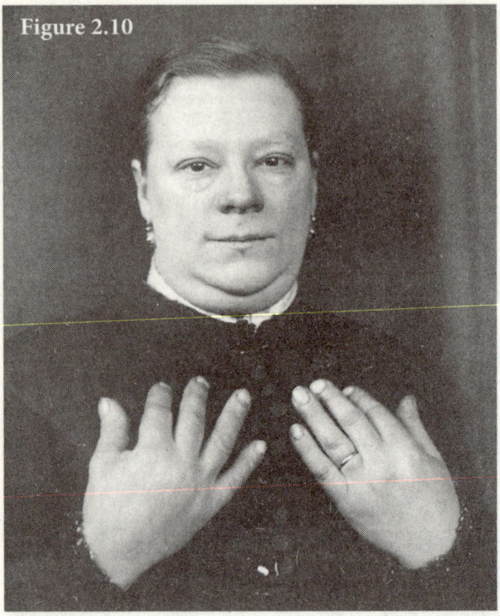

Figure 2.10

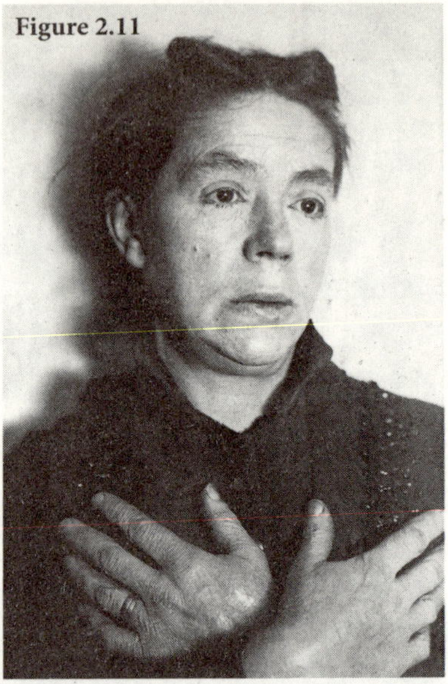

Figure 2.11

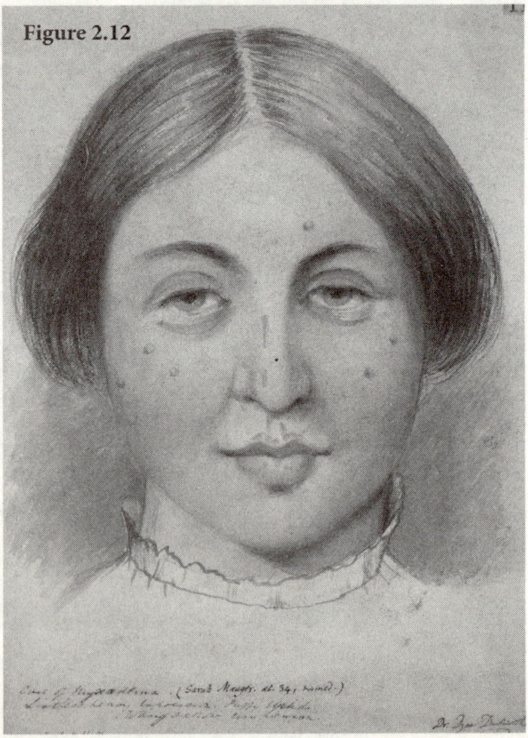

Figure 2.12

Figure 2.10 Photograph of woman showing typical appearances in the face and hands due to myxoedema (hypothyroidism).[16]
St Bartholomew's Hospital Archives and Museum, London.
Credit: Wellcome collection

Figure 2.11 Woman with myxoedema (hypothyroidism) at an early stage.[17]
St Bartholomew's Hospital Archives and Museum, London.
Credit: Wellcome collection

Figure 2.12 Watercolour drawing of the face of a married woman, aged 34 years, affected with myxoedema. The listless expression, puffy eyelids, and waxy complexion, associated with this affection, are well marked.[18]
Credit: Godart, Thomas, Wellcome collection

Figures 2.9 to 2.12 show women suffering from hypothyroidism (myxoedema). Myxoedema is an old name for the same symptoms as hypothyroidism. Myxoedema is mucus oedema. It refers to swelling of skin and fluid build-up in the body, the typical symptoms of hypothyroidism

Blood: In hypothyroidism, there is a reduction in number of one type of white blood cells, called lymphocytes (usually from 30% to 18% of total white blood cells).[14] Lymphocytes fight infections by creating antibodies against bacteria, virus, and other invaders. There is increase in the number of another type of white blood cells, called eosinophils (usually from 2%–3% to 11%–16% of white blood cells).[6] Eosinophils are known for their role in allergy symptoms. They fight parasites, as well as viral and fungal infections.

From the above description of symptoms, we see that in hypothyroidism disease, every organ of the body—bones, muscles, brain, skin, hair, nails—is affected. In fact, in hypothyroidism disease, every cell in the body is affected. This is reflected in symptoms in every organ. The symptoms detailed in cretinism give us an insight into all the possible symptoms in hypothyroidism, although the severity of symptoms is much less in hypothyroidism. As hypothyroidism is a milder form of thyroid disease, only a few organs may be affected. A few people may see symptoms in certain organs, and a few others may see symptoms in certain other organs. It is not necessary that a person suffering from hypothyroidism should show all the above-described symptoms.

References

1. McClelland J. An inquiry into the nature and causes of goitre. In: *Some Inquiries in The Province of Kemaon, Relative to Geology, and Other Branches of Natural Science.* Calcutta: Thacker & Co. and Cantor & Co.; 1835.
2. Woman with large goitre. https://wellcomecollection.org/works/nxqy4m7e/images?id=j9x59qfj. Accessed May 12, 2022.

3. Woman, possibly with goitre. https://wellcomecollection.org/works/d8xuzwpb/images?id=fnj3vb5k. Accessed May 12, 2022.
4. Boy affected with parenchymatous goitre at an early stage. https://wellcomecollection.org/works/anfnkn2y/images?id=agybysqc. Accessed May 12, 2022.
5. Girl with large cystic goitre. https://wellcomecollection.org/works/r5hrwm58/images?id=m5u599wz. Accessed May 12, 2022.
6. Clements FW. Health significance of endemic goitre and related conditions. In: *Endemic Goitre.* Monograph Series No. 44. Geneva: World Health Organization; 1960:246.
7. Beckers C, Benmiloud M. Africa. In: Stanbury JB, Hetzel BS, eds. *Endemic Goiter and Endemic Cretinism*. John Wiley; 1980:76.
8. Wells E. *Essay Upon Cretinism and Goitre.* London: John Churchill; 1845:15-25.
9. Blackie GS. *Cretins and Cretinism,* A Prize Thesis of University of Edinburgh. Edinburgh: Maclachlan & Stewart and London: Simpkin, Marshall & Co.; 1855.
10. Female, non-goitrous cretinism. https://wellcomecollection.org/works/n7qgxmnp/images?id=tduh3jm9. Accessed May 12, 2022.
11. Bramwell B. https://wellcomecollection.org/works/tqrxax48/images?id=kb2qjkcy. Accessed May 12, 2022.
12. Bramwell B. https://wellcomecollection.org/works/tqrxax48/images?id=nc6d8hgu. Accessed May 12, 2022.
13. Male sporadic cretin. https://wellcomecollection.org/works/rpq5s49s/images?id=e4z4rrnn. Accessed May 12, 2022.
14. Kocher ET. Concerning pathological manifestations in low-grade thyroid diseases, Nobel Lecture, December 11, 1909. Nobelprize.org. https://www.nobelprize.org/uploads/2018/06/kocher-lecture.pdf. Accessed: May 8, 2022.

15. The face and hands of a woman, aged 47, suffering from well-marked myxoedema. https://wellcomecollection.org/works/bjd6vfr6 Accessed May 12, 2022.

16. Typical appearances in the face and hands due to myxoedema. https://wellcomecollection.org/works/qsz7gewq. Accessed May 12, 2022.

17. Woman with myxoedema at an early stage. https://wellcomecollection.org/works/r7s6fzzr/images?id=hycvyctu. Accessed May 12, 2022.

18. Face of a woman affected with myxoedema. https://wellcomecollection.org/works/fthkgqcn. Accessed May 12, 2022.

Chapter 3

Geographical Distribution of Goiter and Cretinism

In this chapter, we will look at the geographic locations where goiter and cretinism were most prevalent in the past. This will give us a clue to *the cause* of thyroid disease.

i. Europe

In Europe, the Alps Mountain range was the epicenter of *endemic* goiter. A disease is said to be endemic in a region if 10% or more of the population has the disease. The Alps Mountain range is primarily spread across four countries, Switzerland, Austria, Italy, and France. In Switzerland and Austria, the majority of the country is covered with the Alps, and it is in these two countries that the highest incidence of goiter and cretinism was observed in the past.

Country-specific research on goiter and cretinism detailed below, unless specified, is adapted from a paper written by Kelly and Snedden for the World Health Organization (WHO) in 1960.[1] The paper was part of a monograph series published by WHO on endemic goiter.[2] When other sources are quoted, separate citations are provided below.

Switzerland

Practically, all parts of Switzerland were prone to goiter. In many localities, the disease was associated with mental deficiency, deaf-mutism, and other body/mind disorders. Switzerland is divided into 26 cantons. A canton is similar to a state in other countries. The incidence of goiter was severe in almost all the cantons. However, there was less goiter in the north-western cantons of Basel, Solothurn, and Neuchâtel, i.e., in the cantons less covered with the Alps mountains. About 1838, it was noted that the use of waters from certain sources (Department Léman in the hamlet of Thuet) produced goiter in 8 or 10 days.[3]

In 1920, in one of the most severely affected cantons, the canton of Valais, a survey among school children showed that about 70% of them had goiter. A note must be made here about the statistics relating to goiter. Within the canton of Valais, there may have been areas with 100% goiter prevalence rates and areas with only 50% prevalence rates. The goiter prevalence varied quite widely within short distances. Therefore, there is not much meaning we can draw from goiter prevalence statistics of a whole country or a state. The goiter prevalence of a *specific locality* is what matters to understand *the cause* of thyroid disease. We will go through such an analysis in the next chapter, where we will analyze goiter prevalence statistics locality by locality over short distances of about one to two miles. In this chapter, we will restrict ourselves to getting a broad overview of the geographies where goiter and cretinism were most prevalent.

Switzerland was also the center of the most severe form of thyroid disease—cretinism. About the year 1850, out of the total Switzerland population of 2 million, no less than 20,000 persons were estimated to have suffered from cretinism.[4] This would mean that approximately 1% of the Swiss population suffered from the most severe form of thyroid disease.

The following was the prevalence rate of cretinism in various cantons of Switzerland according to a report published in 1855.[4(p10)] Table 3.1 on the next page shows that in Valais and de Vaud, cretinism was a common malady.

Table 3.1 Prevalence of Cretinism in Switzerland

Canton	Prevalence rate of cretinism
Valais	1 in 25 inhabitants
de Vaud	1 in 27 inhabitants
Uri	1 in 83 inhabitants
Argovie	1 in 167 inhabitants
Grisons	1 in 266 inhabitants
Glarus	1 in 375 inhabitants

Austria

Just as in Switzerland, in the past, almost all parts of Austria were severely affected by goiter. The areas free of goiter were the areas where the Alps mountains were not present. In 1923–24, in a survey of 700,000 school children, about 44% of boys and 48% of girls were found to be goitrous.

Austria, just like Switzerland, had very high number of cretins. Along the banks of the river Danube in Upper Austria, the disease was so universal that whole families consisted of only cretins and half cretins—and to such an extent, that in villages of four to five thousand inhabitants, not one man was capable of bearing arms. The prevalence of cretinism in the different provinces of Austria is indicated in Table 3.2.[4(p11)]

Table 3.2 Prevalence of Cretinism in Austria

Province	Prevalence rate of cretinism
Judenburg	1 in 53 inhabitants
Bruck	1 in 74 inhabitants
Gratz	1 in 150 inhabitants
Marburg	1 in 374 inhabitants
Cilly	1 in 516 inhabitants

Italy

There are many descriptions of goiter and cretinism in the classics of Italian literature. Italian literature of the Middle Ages shows that thyroid disease was a problem in Italy from the earliest times.

Geographically, high goiter rates occurred to a varying degree throughout the whole of the Alps Mountain range region in north Italy. This disease also occurred in the north and south plains of the river Po, although the disease was much less severe than that in the Alps region in north Italy. Investigations in 1920–1938 indicated that in the area between the Alps and the river Po, thyroid enlargement was found in 20–30% of school children. In the high mountain district, these figures rose to 50%–60%. In certain communities, it reached 70%–80%. Indeed, rates of 100% were also common. Goiter also occurred in the Ligurian Apennines, a mountain range in northwestern Italy, immediately north of Genoa, a port city in northwest Italy.

The royal survey of Sardinia showed that around 1850, in the population of 4 million, no less than 10,000 people were estimated to be cretins.[4(p11)] In 1883, in the provinces of Piedmont, Lombardy, and Venice, one in every 67 inhabitants was either goitrous or a cretin.

France

The geographical distribution of goiter in France was in the following principal mountainous zones. Goiter, in the eastern belt, extended along the entire German–Swiss–Italian border from northern Alsace to the Alps-Maritimes on the Mediterranean coast. Goiter was also prevalent in the Auvergne and Massif Central, the south-central regions of France within mountainous landscape.

The heaviest intensity of goiter was in Savoy, the southeastern end of France, where the Tarentaise and Maurienne mountain ranges were intersected by many goitrous valleys. The essential cause of goiter was regarded as the water in this area. There existed "conscript springs", where military recruits used to go to drink the water in order to develop neck swelling and so escape military service. At a boarding school in St. Jean-de-Maurienne, the students developed goiters during term but lost them when on holiday out of this area, only to develop them again on returning to school. "Holiday" goiter developed rapidly in individuals from other parts of the country who chose to spend their vacation in these "goiter districts."

Cretinism in France was recorded in Savoy, Maurienne, and Vosages. In 1874, Baillarger noted that there were, in France alone, no less than half a million goitrous persons and 122,700 cretins. Records of goiter among domestic animals are occasionally met with in the French literature. In 1862, Baillarger described occurrences of goiter among mules, horses, and dogs in the mountainous eastern part of France.

Germany

In 1975, an extensive study of goiter prevalence in 5.4 million military conscripts was published. About 15% of them had goiter.[5]

In Germany, the goiter belt ran along the mountain ranges in the country. There were five main goiter zones. One extended from the spa town of Baden-Baden in West Germany near the borders of France, through the mountains of Breisgau and the Black-Forest, eastward through Württemberg (the area around present-day city of Stuttgart) and southern Bavaria, to the Austrian borders. The second extended from Vogtland in eastern Germany, near the borders of Czech Republic, to Erzgebirge. The third extended from the borders of Luxembourg, north-eastward along the Hunsrück and Taunus ridges, through Hesse and Lower Franconia into Thruringia, a state in central Germany. The fourth comprised Münsterland of northwestern Germany and parts of Westphalia. The fifth belt occurred in Brandenburg, extending from the region of Cottbus south-eastward into Polish Silesia.

Cretinism was endemic in various parts of Rhenish Prussia, the area of present-day western Germany, along the lower Rhine River. An island named Niederwörth in the Rhine, a mile and a half below the city of Coblence, was a remarkable example. On this small island, no fewer than 40 among 750 inhabitants were found to be cretins.[4(p11)] In the vicinity of the Lake of Laach, near Bonn, there were many cretins in all stages; and in one of the villages of the district, there were 22 cretins among 300 inhabitants. In the Grand Duchy of Baden, the report of the Sanitary Commission of 1847 mentioned the existence of 490 cretins, chiefly in the Black Forest and the Odenwald.[4(p11)] In Bavaria in Lower Franconia, in half a million inhabitants, there were, according to Professor Virchow, at least 200 cretins. In Württemberg, it was calculated that there were about 5,000 people affected by the disease. In highlands of Bavaria, the disease was common, although not statistically reported.[4(p11)]

Spain

There was great deal of goiter in Spain. Almost all mountainous districts were affected, but few of them were affected to a serious degree.

Las Hurdes, a region in western Spain, bordering Portugal, constituted an incomparable field for the study of goiter. It was the focus point in all of Spain. The area is composed of three long narrow valleys of unbelievably rough and inhospitable country. The prevalence of goiter exceeded 25%, and the large numbers of the goitrous population also had symptoms of cretinism. Cases of idiotism, deaf-mutism, and dwarfism were many, and not a single man from the district was found fit for military service.

In northern Spain, a belt of very considerable intensity extended from Catalonia, along the Pyrenees Mountain range, through the Cantabrian Mountains range (one of the main mountain ranges in Spain) and the Asturias (a region of northwest Spain, known for its rugged coast and mountains), to the Galicia (the region above Portugal) in the West. The Pyrenees Mountain range forms a wall between Spain and France.

In central Spain, goiter was found along the Sierra Gredos Mountain range in the south of Avila Province west of Madrid.

In southern Spain, the most goitrous province was Granada, where the region of Las Alpujarras on the southward slopes of the Sierra Nevada (a mountain range in southern Spain) was highly affected.

We may note that all the goitrous regions in Spain were located in and around the mountainous regions.

England and Wales

In 1924, an all-England survey of 375,000 school children was undertaken by the medical department of the Board of Education. The survey revealed that among school children of 12 years age, the goiter rate was

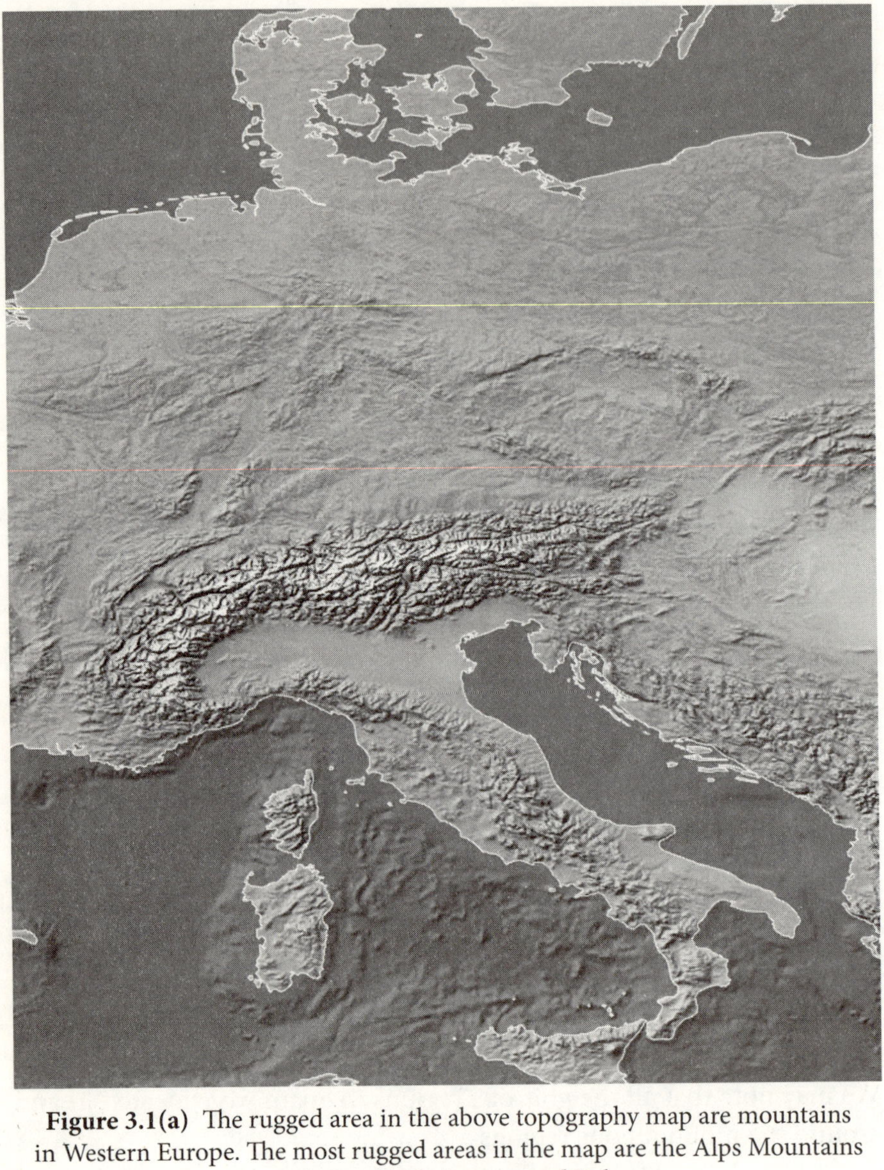

Figure 3.1(a) The rugged area in the above topography map are mountains in Western Europe. The most rugged areas in the map are the Alps Mountains in Switzerland, Austria, and Italy.

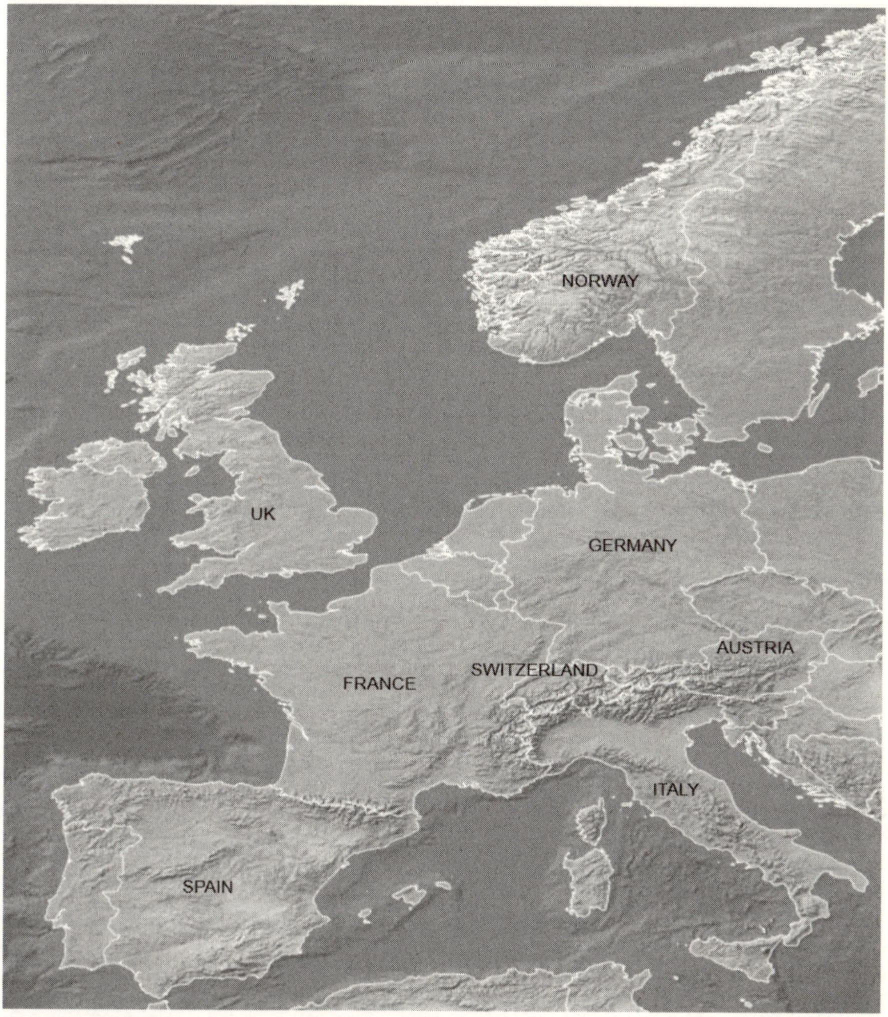

Figure 3.1(b) The topography of Western Europe with country labels. The rugged areas are mountainous regions.

5% in boys and 13% in girls in areas of high prevalence, and 1% in boys and 4% in girls in areas of low prevalence. But in some places, notably Devon, Somerset, Oxfordshire, Northumberland, and Durham, the goiter rates were 10%–20% among boys and more than 30% among girls. "Derbyshire neck" branded the Derbyshire County as goitrous, albeit unfairly, for goiter was equally severe, if not more so in Oxfordshire, Gloucestershire, Somerset, and Dorset.

Greece

About 80% of Greece consists of mountains or hills, making the country one of the most mountainous in Europe. In 1948, a clinical examination of 12,000 children and youth disclosed a goiter rate of 53% in an appreciable number of villages in the northern districts of Greece.

Poland

Practically the whole of the south Poland was goitrous. The individuals who migrated from a goiter-free district to live in Lower Silesia, a goiter-prone district, were also known to develop goiter.

ii. North America

United States of America

From east to west, the "goiter centers" of United States were found through the length of the Appalachian Mountain range, the states bordering the Great Lakes, North Dakota, and into the far west states of Montana, Idaho, Utah, Oregon, and Washington, where the incidence was particularly heavy. Except for isolated pockets of high incidence in Kansas and in the New Orleans district of Louisiana, the great central plains were comparatively goiter-free. Similarly, the states on the Atlantic seaboard and the southern states of Mississippi, Alabama, Georgia, and Florida were comparatively goiter-free.

The first reliable index of the over-all prevalence of goiter in the United States was from the examination of 2.5 million men drafted for military service during the First World War, between 1914 and 1918. Nearly, 12,000 men had simple goiter, and 31% of these men were rejected. The frequency of the disease was greatest among recruits from the states of Washington, Oregon, Montana, and Idaho in the northwest and from the region of the Great Lakes. It was least in men drafted from the southern and Atlantic coast states and was most frequently seen in those of Scandinavian origin.

Between 1923 and 1929, systematic goiter surveys of elementary school children were made in various states by the US Public Health Service. The results revealed a general distribution very much similar to the above military survey, except that whereas the examination of drafted men disclosed the highest incidence in the states of the Pacific Northwest, the surveys of the Public Health Service indicated the greatest incidence to be in certain areas of the Midwest, that is, in states grouped around the Great Lakes—Ohio, Indiana, Illinois, Michigan, Iowa, Wisconsin, and Minnesota. In the town of Cincinnati, Ohio, for example, 26% of the boys and 40% of the girls had goiter. In Minnesota, the endemic was more serve, with 41% of boys and 70% of girls from 13 different localities showing evidence of thyroid enlargement. Conditions in Michigan and Wisconsin were no better; rates of 40%, 60%, 70%, and even 100% were reported among boys and girls from certain localities in these states.

Throughout the eastern states, although some moderately high percentages were recorded by the US Public Health Service, there was, on the whole, much less goiter than that around the Great Lakes and in the far West. The State of Connecticut had goiter rates of 7% in boys and 29% in girls, and Massachusetts had goiter rates of 9% in boys and 22% in girls.

As regards the far West, in Colorado, thyroid enlargement was 25% in boys and 30% in girls. Utah was a notoriously goitrous state, with very high rates found in the locality of Salt Lake City. In Oregon, thyroid enlargement was noted in 22% of boys and 38% of girls. Goiter was endemic to a considerable extent in the coastal towns of Oregon, indicating that proximity to the sea did not necessarily guarantee freedom from the disease.

In short, goiter, a severe form of thyroid disease, was prevalent across the country. At present, hypothyroidism in the United States likely shares a similar geography.

Canada

Travelling from west to east, in the past, goiter was noted across Canada. In the western-most province of Canada, there were centers of goiter in British Columbia. About 60 miles from Vancouver, the largest city in British Columbia, the disease was found in the Pemberton Valley and in the area watered by the Lillooet and Birkenhead rivers. About 1915, European settlers in Pemberton Meadows suffered so severely from goiter, both in themselves and among their cattle, pigs, and horses, that they almost decided to leave the valley. The coastal valley of Bella Coola, 270 miles northwest of Vancouver, was also affected. Other areas with considerable prevalence in British Columbia were to the east and the northeast of Vancouver. To the north there were goiter centers in the Cariboo Mountains, at the town of Prince George, and all along the Grand Trunk Pacific Railway, as far as Edmonton.

Edmonton is the capital city of Alberta province in West Canada. There was a great deal of goiter in Edmonton, located north of Saskatchewan River, to the northern border of the United States. Another part of Alberta where goiter was common was the area to the northwest of Edmonton, in the area drained by the upper waters of the Peace and Athabasca rivers. Most of the affected parts of the Alberta landscape encompassed mountains. Between 1819 and 1822, an early account of goiter in this area was given by Dr. John Richardson, a Scottish surgeon and scientist on John Franklin's famous expedition to the polar seas. "At Edmonton," he noted "the disorder attacks only those who drink the water of the North Saskatchewan River. The inhabitants of Rocky Mountain House, 60 miles nearer the source of the river, are more severely affected than those of Edmonton; but at Carlton House, a considerable distance below Edmonton, the disease is known only by name. A residence of a single year at Edmonton is sufficient to render a family goitrous."

In Saskatchewan, a province to the east of Alberta, there were accounts of goiter at Saskatoon. In 1934, the prevalence of goiter among school children here was estimated at 12%.

In Manitoba, a province to the east of Saskatchewan, goiter studies of school children were made at widely separated places. At Dauphine, in the west of the province, 74% of children were affected, while at Morden, in the south, 21% of children had goiter. At Winnipeg, the goiter rate was 50%. In the towns of Birds Hill and Stonewall, 85% of the children suffered from goiter.

Further east from the Manitoba province, the area surrounding the five Great Lakes was recognized as notoriously goitrous for a long time. Goiter was also observed in the Japanese Prisoners of War Camp at Angler on the north shore of Lake Superior.

Mexico

The Rio Grande is one of the principal rivers of the southwestern United States and northern Mexico. The upper basin of this river was a great goiter zone.

According to Stacpoole, the greatest authority on goiter in Mexico, endemic centers were found in all Mexican states bordering the Pacific, except lower California. Goiter also affected the midcentral and southern parts of the country. The northcentral gulf-coast of Tamaulipas and the Caribbean regions of Campeche, Yucatan, and Quintana Roo were practically exempt. Most of the goiter centers were situated in the mountains, but there were also stretches along the Pacific coast where the disease was found.

Up to the end of 1952, Stacpoole and his colleagues examined more than one million children and adults in eight midcentral states with a total population of over 10 million. The survey covered 3,756 towns and villages within 858 townships. The results of the survey indicated that in these eight states, there were more than two million people afflicted with goiter, i.e., 20% of the population was affected. Goiter rates of more than 80% were common in many places, and in some communities, goiter rates were upward of 90%.

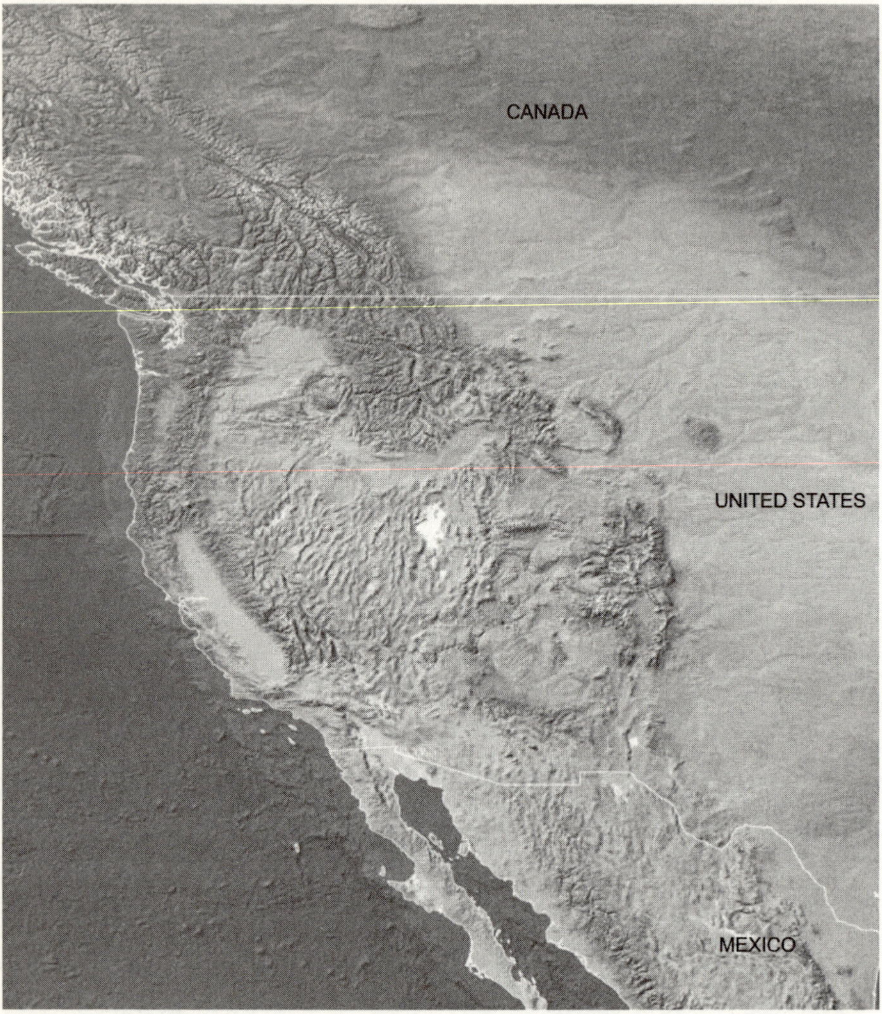

Figure 3.2(a) The topography of Western Canada, Western USA and Mexico. The rugged areas are mountainous regions.
Copyright: EUMETSAT

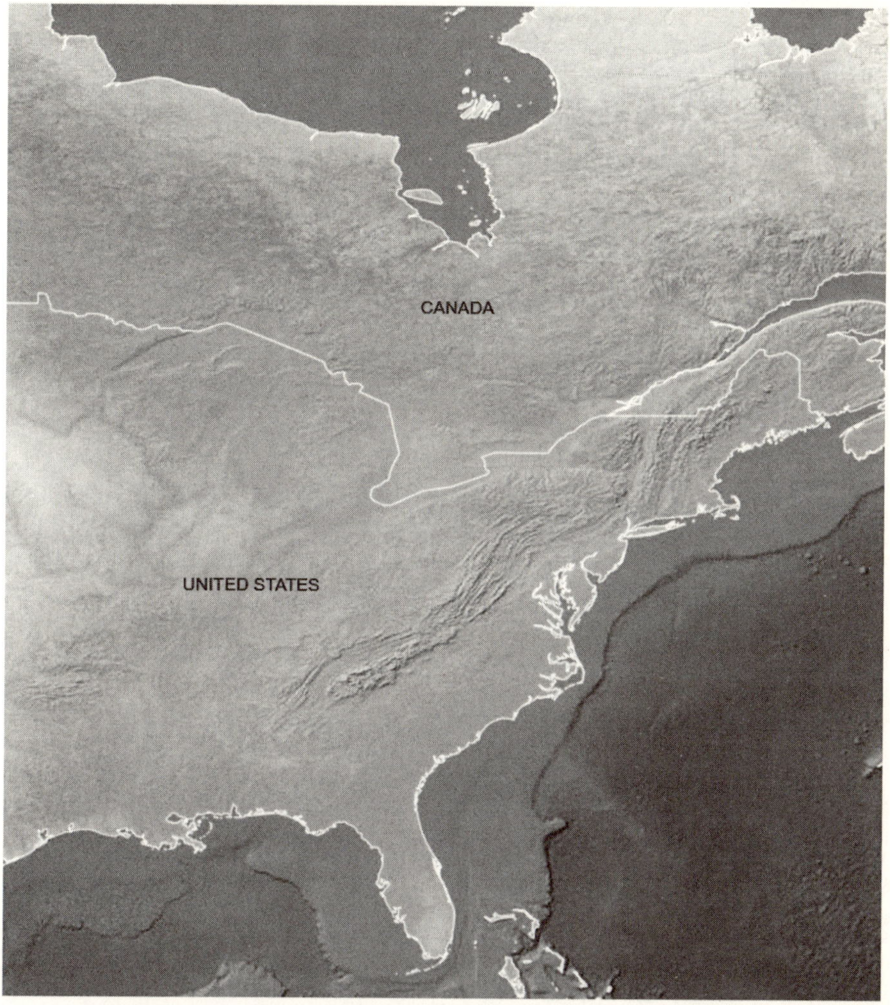

Figure 3.2(b) The topography of Eastern Canada and Eastern USA. It is less rugged than Western USA.
Copyright: EUMETSAT

iii. South America

Colombia

The first explorers of Colombia were astonished to find the banks of the Magdalena River inhabited by a race of "heavy and stupid savages of sluggish habit who passed their days in sleep."

Endemic goiter in Colombia was a problem of long standing. In 1760, goiter was reported on the upper Magdalena River. In 1810, it was observed that goiter was frequent in the convents of Bogota, where well-water of exceptional hardness was used for drinking and cooking purposes.

In 1942, about 10% of 153,000 prospective recruits for military service examined over a period of five years were rejected because of simple goiter. In 1945, the Department of Nutrition of the Cooperative Health Service began a four-year survey of the geographical distribution and frequency of simple goiter among school children aged 7–14 throughout the country. Few, if any, complete surveys of this kind were ever made anywhere in the world. They covered 183,243 children in 14 departments, and the analysis showed an average goiter rate of 53%, the highest being 81% in the Department of Caldas. Another interesting conclusion drawn from the survey was that in places with soft or semihard water, the goiter incidence was less than those in places with hard or very hard water. Where the endemic was of long duration (100 years or more), the physique of the people was substandard, and there was evidence of cretinism and retarded mental development.

There is a special interest to the story of goiter in Colombia because it was here that the famous French scientist J. B. Boussingault put forward for the first time, in 1831, the recommendation that domestic salt supplies should be iodized to prevent goiter. The circumstances of this recommendation were that in 1824, von Humboldt described the occurrence of goiter in the Andean plateau and referred to the striking fact that the inhabitants of goitrous localities recognized that salt from certain natural deposits was more beneficial than that from others. On analysis, Boussingault found that the salts instinctively preferred by the goitrous people contained the highest iodine. This prompted Boussingault to recommend iodized salt for goiter.

Argentina

In Argentina, the highest goiter rates were in the provinces and territories bordering the eastern slope of the Cordillera mountains. In this vast, 1500-mile strip of territory, goiter was known since the Spanish conquest. In 1820, writing of Mendoza Province, Schmidtmeyer observed, "The greatest number of the inhabitants of this state were afflicted with that unseemly and injurious disorder, the goiter." In 1931, in some departments of Jujuy, a goiter rate of 100 % was observed. In a 1937 census of schools in 16 different places in Mendoza, goiter rates varied from 28% to 88 % among children, the average rate being 44%. In 1938, in San Pedrito, a 77% goiter rate was noted in school children. Salta was no less goitrous. In Tucuman, rates of 65 % in boys and 60 % in girls were recorded, and the 1938 survey disclosed an average rate of 23% for the whole province.

Uruguay

In 1935, an important observation was made in Uruguay. The thyroid glands of human subjects, cattle, and dogs examined *postmortem* (i.e., after death), showed a normal iodine content. On the other hand, determinations of the calcium content of normal and diseased human thyroid glands showed that hypothyroid glands had high calcium levels, whereas hyperthyroid glands had a low calcium content.

Brazil

Endemic goiter was a problem of exceptional gravity in parts of Brazil. The disease was particularly rampant in the southern states of Rio Grande, Santa Catarina, Parana, and Sao Paulo, the southeastern states of Rio de Janeiro and Minas Gerais, and the great central and western states of Goias and Mato Grosso. In the north and northeastern parts of the country, goiter was less noticeable.

Between 1940 and 1947, a study of endemic goiter examined 22,000 infants, school children, and college students in different parts of the

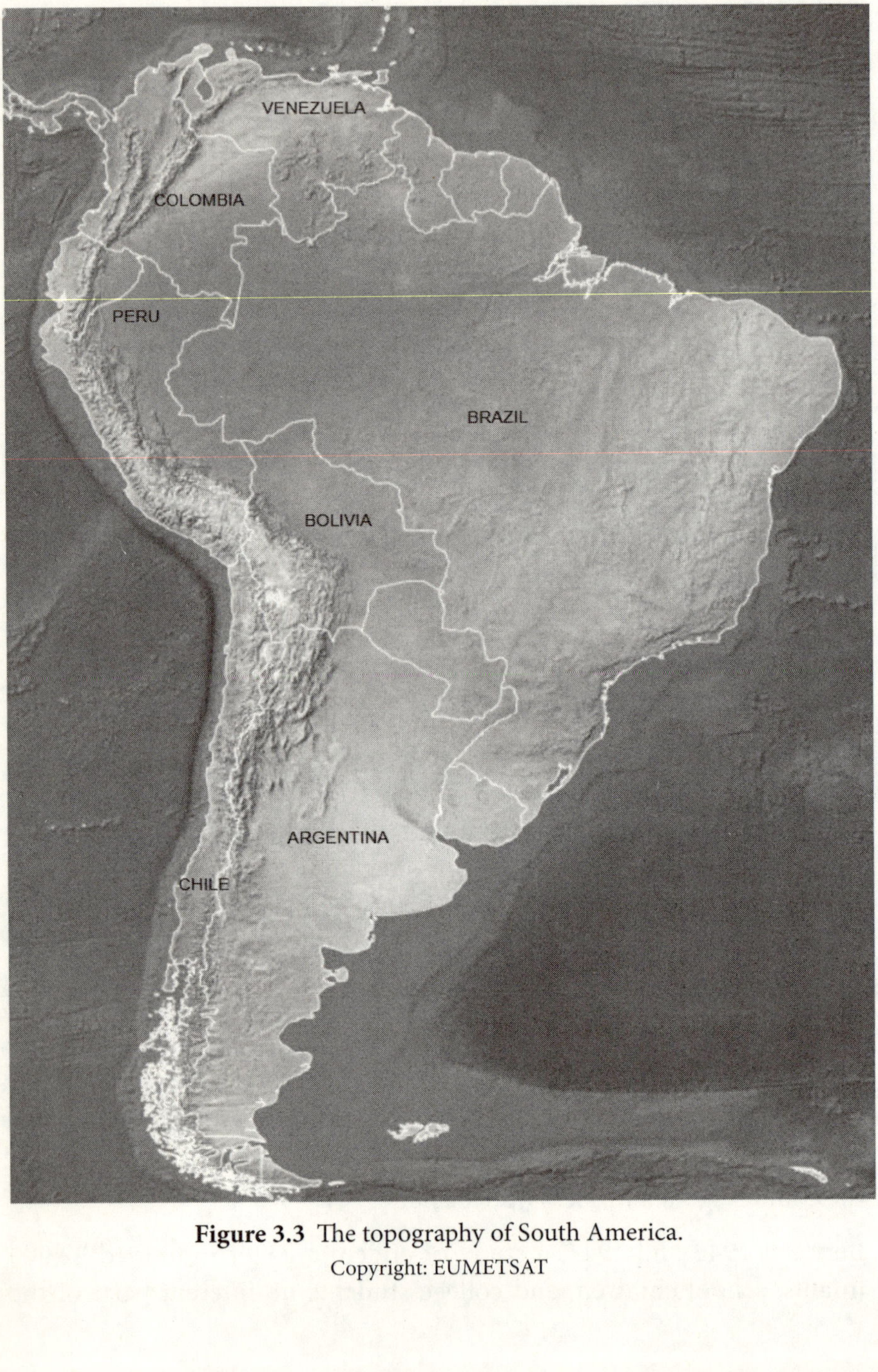

Figure 3.3 The topography of South America.
Copyright: EUMETSAT

state of Sao Paulo and found goiter rates of 5%–10% in coastal districts, gradually increasing through the valley of the Parahiba river into the highlands of the interior, where goiter rates of 60%, 70%, and even 90% were encountered along the Serra da Mantiqueira, a mountain range in southeastern Brazil, which dominates the hinterland between the cities of Sao Paulo and Rio de Janeiro.

About 1940, Duarte Nunes reported that physical incapacity due to thyroid insufficiency was of frequent occurrence among army recruits examined by him in the military hospital at Curitiba, the capital of the southern Brazilian state of Paraná. Men with goiters were indolent, lazy and easily tired. After physical effort, tremor of the limbs was a marked feature. For these reasons Duarte Nunes recommended that anyone suffering from goiter be excluded from the Brazilian army. In 1955, this matter was reexamined in great detail. Inspection of more than 120,000 young men of military age (19–20 years), drawn from nearly 200 municipalities in the states of Parana, Santa Catarina, and Rio Grande do Sul revealed that 50%–80% of recruits were rejected for service on account of ill-health and physical disability, and among the causes of rejection, goiter stood high, with goiter rates of 25% common in the upland areas of southern Brazil.

So great was the intensity of the endemic in the interior of the State of Rio de Janeiro that nearly all the inhabitants were affected and any person without goiter was regarded as abnormal.

iv. Asia

India

In Asia, the highest incidence of goiter and cretinism was in the Himalayan Mountain range. The Himalayan Mountain range forms the northern physical border of India. The Himalayan Mountain range passes through Pakistan, India, Bhutan, and Nepal. The Himalayas are home to the highest mountain peaks in the world. The world's highest mountain, Mount Everest, is in the Himalayas. More than one hundred mountain peaks have an altitude over 23,600 feet. By comparison, the highest peak outside Asia has an altitude of 22,838 ft (Aconcagua, in the Andes).[6]

It was at the foothills of the Himalayan Mountains that the severe forms of thyroid disease, goiter and cretinism were widely observed. It was also here that the finest research on thyroid disease was done by the British medical doctors John McClelland and Robert McCarrison. For more than 1500 miles along the Himalayas, the intensity of the disease was so great in some places as to merit the term superendemic.[7] The goiter belt ran along all the Indian states bordering the Himalayan Mountains. Cretinism and deaf-mutism were also common in these states. These diseases were prevalent only in the mountainous parts of the states; the plain areas of the states were less affected.

In Central India, goiter was common along the Vindhya and the Satpura mountain ranges and along the Narmada River, which flows between these two mountain ranges. In the central Indian plateau, goiter was found in the neighborhood of the southern tributaries of the Yamuna River and in the Jhansi–Lalitpur uplands, where these river tributaries originate. There were also reports of goiter in Surguja district (in Chhattisgarh state), Ranchi district (in Jharkhand state), and Sambalpur (in Orissa state).

In South India, goiter was prevalent in the regions along the Eastern Ghat and Western Ghat mountains. Eastern Ghats and Western Ghats are the mountain ranges along the East coast and West coast of India respectively. Robert McCarrison observed that "Madras side and the Eastern Ghats are practically free of goiter." But I know from my personal observation in the Eastern Ghats, where my hometown is located, that goiter occurs here even today. This shows that even a stalwart researcher like McCarrison cannot give a comprehensive description of goiter geography as the incidence of the disease varies widely over short distances.

Cretinism and Deaf-Mutism in India

The heavily affected areas of cretinism, deaf-mutism, and idiocy were located at the foothills of the Himalayas. In these areas, the average rate of goiter was 40%, and the rate of deaf-mutism was 4%.[8] The number of deaf-mutes in the age group of 0–5 years was vastly underestimated because the parents hesitated to report their children as defective until all hope was lost, clinging as long as possible to the belief that speech and hearing were merely delayed.

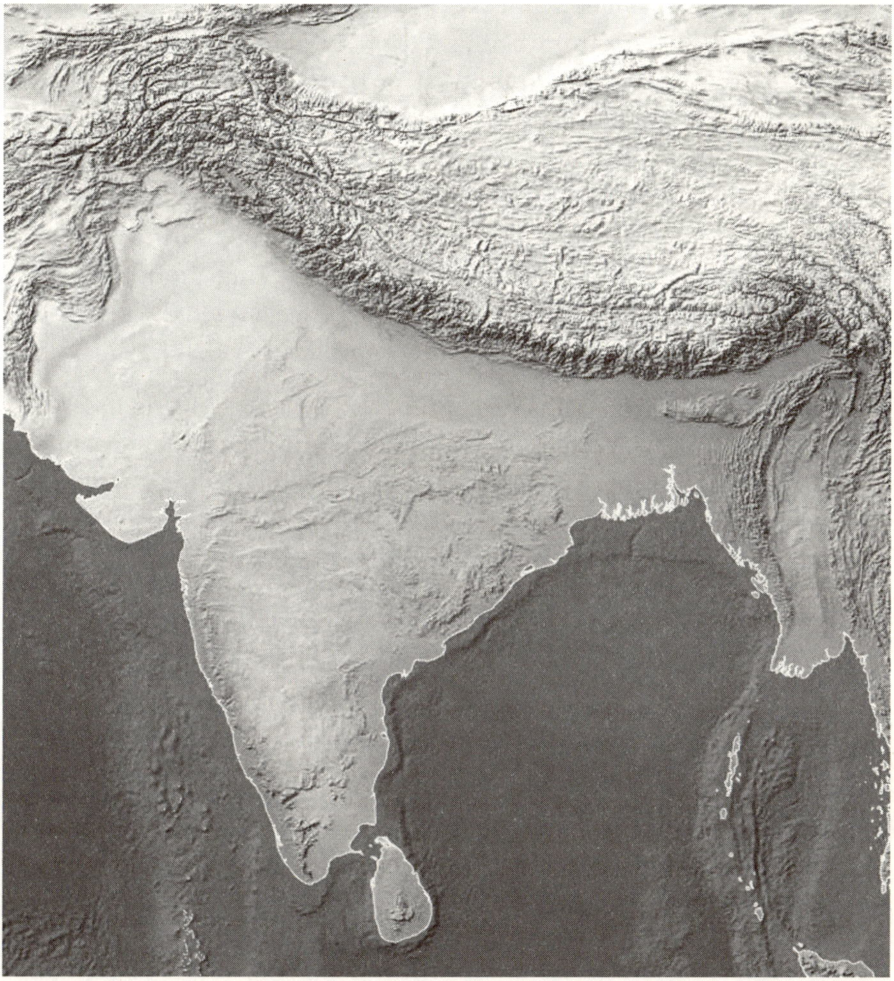

Figure 3.4 The topography of India.
The very rugged area in the north are the Himalayas.
Copyright: EUMETSAT

China

A significant portion of China's land area is covered with mountains. Mountains, plateaus, and hills account for 70% of China's land surface.[9] As a rule, endemic goiter and cretinism were prominent in mountainous areas in China.[10]

Endemic goiter is of ancient lineage in China. Most of the earliest written records of goiter were from China. From times immemorial, travelers into the North, West, and Southwest provinces of China were struck by the human degradation caused by goiter and cretinism; their diaries and journals were full of vivid impressions of these scenes. Around the year 1275, Marco Polo, the famous traveler from Venice in Italy to the court of the Grand Khan in China, saw goiters in the Chinese Turkestan provinces of Kashgar and Yarkand. Writing about the people of Yarkand, Marco Polo said, "They are in general afflicted with tumors in the throat, occasioned by the quality of water they drink."

The map in Figure 3.5 helps us recognize the names of provinces that we will discuss in the goiter-description of China. The imaginary line in the map divides China into two parts. About 94% of China's population lives to the right of line and about 6% lives to left of the line.[13] The land area to the left of the line is the most mountainous and inhospitable part of China, and hence the low population in the region.

Endemic goiter was reported from all provinces and cities, except Shanghai. According to various researchers in China, the incidence of goiter varied from 20% to 60%, depending on the locality.[10] This was based on research conducted between 1910 and 1979 by various researchers in seven provinces, namely, Hubei, Ningxia, Anhui, Tianjin, Guizhou, Hebei, and Yunnan.[10] Cretinism in China was equally widespread. The incidence of cretinism varied from 0.5% to 3% of the population. In one exceptional locality in the San-Jian plains, Northeast China, cretinism was noted in 11% of the population.

Goiter Belt Covered Almost Entire China

The goiter belt of China began in the northeast near Shanhaiguan in Hebei Province on the southern border of the Northeast Administrative

Area of China, previously known as Manchuria; it followed a westward semicircular route across the mountainous watershed, north of Beijing, into Eastern Inner Mongolia, and then turned south through the Province of Gansu, as far as Qinghai. From there, it extended through Sikang and the western regions of Sichuan and Guizhou into Yunnan, the most goitrous province in all of China. With the possible exception of Chongming Island, at the mouth of the Yangtse river, where goiter was noted by Maxwell, all the coastal provinces, including those of the great plains in the East and Center of China, were virtually goiter-free, at least so far as the simple endemic variety was concerned; but

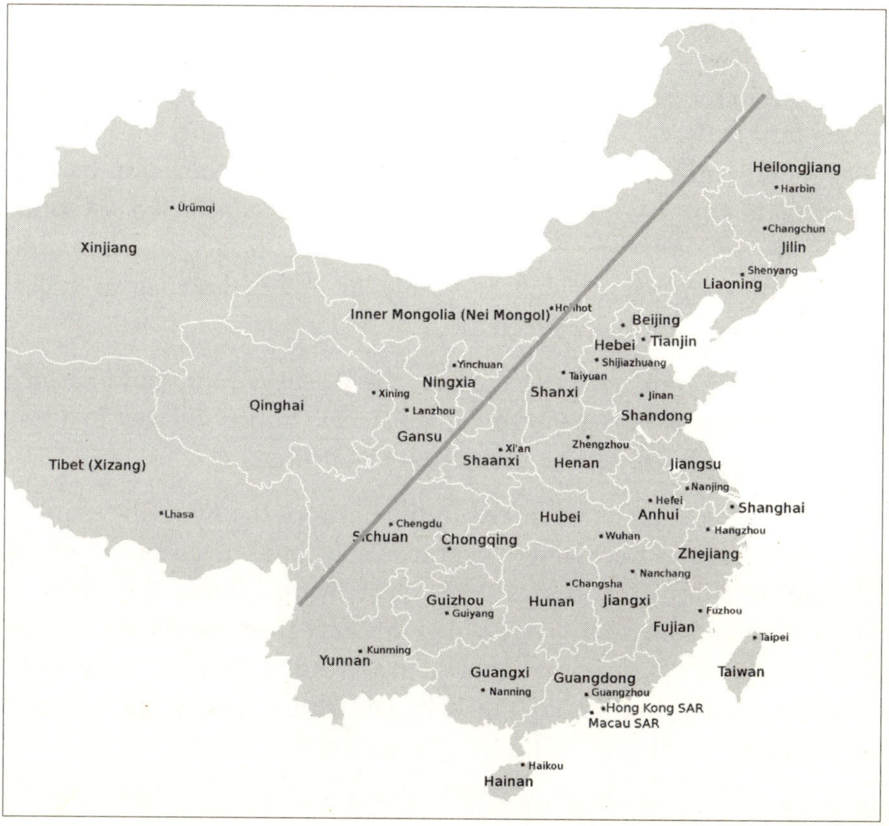

Figure 3.5 Provinces of China. Map (Author: Sameboat);[11] Imaginary line across the map (Author: Stefan Lew, modified by dbslkc).[12]

everywhere in these provinces, cases of hyperthyroidism were frequent. Thus, while a few researchers have noted that only Shanghai was free from goiter, a few others noted that the all the coastal provinces and the great plains in East and Central China were free from goiter.

North and Northeast China

The principal focus was Chengde, adjoining Hubei in North China. The endemic here may be regarded as continuous with that occurring along the Great Wall, north of Beijing. Goiter was also severe farther to the north and northwest. The goiter prevalent in Chengde was classified as belonging to the Alpine type (like in the Swiss Alps), and was commonly associated with deaf-mutism, idiocy, cretinism, and myxoedema. The goiter rate varied between 10% and 60%, and in some places, was as high as 85%, as in the Pingchuan area. Chinese and Mongolians were equally prone to the disease, and immigrant Japanese rapidly became victims; a Japanese noncommissioned officer acquired goiter four months after entering the country, and a consular police official contracted a second-degree thyroid enlargement within nine months of being stationed at Pingchuan. As usual, incidence was higher in females than in males; infants were occasionally affected.

The intensity of goiter was severe near the Western Tombs and Eastern Tombs (Imperial Burial Grounds) in Hebei. Entire villages in these regions were reported to be almost 100% goitrous.

East of Chengde, goiter occurred in the basin of the Liao River and in the upland parts of the Liaodong peninsula, where Xiuyan and Huanren Manchu autonomous counties were especially mentioned. Elsewhere in former Manchuria, there were goiter pockets throughout the eastern hills. Other centers were found at Hulan and Suihua, immediately north of Harbin, and throughout the Khingan Mountains in the extreme north, at the headwaters of the Nenjiang river.

West China

During his several expeditions through the Provinces of Gansu, Sichuan, Guizhou, and Yunnan in western China, Hosie saw goiter at many places, in both sexes, and at all ages. Kingrno confirmed that parts of Gansu, particularly the high plateau south of the Mongolian border watered by the upper reaches of the Yellow River, were very goitrous. The disease was also prevalent in the Gold River district on the China–Tibetan border.

Hosie spoke of the enormous goiters he encountered when journeying through the Provinces of Sichuan, Guizhou, and Yunnan in Western China. Warwick made similar references to the prevalence of goiter in many sections of the Great Wall, along which he explored for a thousand miles in the early 1920s. Other western writers recounted similar experiences in different parts of China.

The most impressive accounts of goiter in Yunnan are those by Jeanselme and Robertson. The former entered Yunnan from the south, after completing his goiter survey of Southeast Asian countries (Vietnam and Laos) and saw many cases in the villages and marketplaces frequented by the mountain-dwellers between Manhao, on the southern border, and Kunming, in Yunnan province. Jeanselme estimated the overall goiter rate in Kunming to be about 20%. At Dali, and all around the Great Lake (on which Dali was situated), Jeanselme saw many myxoedematous cretins with puffy faces and unsteady gait.

Robertson's survey some thirty years later, about 1940, revealed that conditions were no different. He was concerned chiefly with the health status of people living along the route of the great Myanmar–China highway and in the adjoining country. Inspection of the adult population working in labor gangs during the construction of the road disclosed a goiter rate of 80% in some gangs; the average in all gangs was over 50%. Robertson was struck by the patchy distribution of the Yunnan endemic. In the northwest, people all along the valleys of the Salween, Mekong, and upper Yangtse rivers were very heavily affected, but the disease was not so evident west of Baoshan. Similarly, on the road from Kunming to Hwei-Tsheh in the northeast, there were villages in which almost everybody had goiter, whereas Hwei-Tsheh itself was not markedly goitrous.

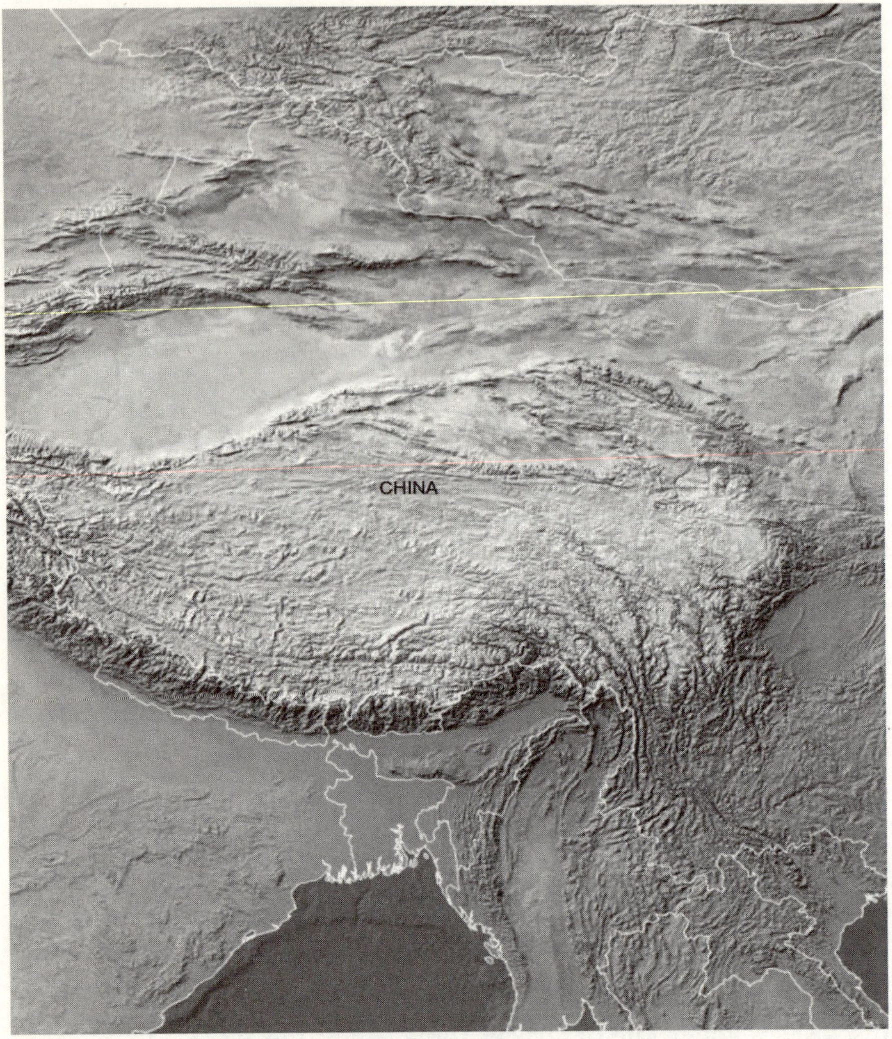

Figure 3.6 The topography of Western China.
Copyright: EUMETSAT

South China

Jeanselme refers to Simon's observation of goiter among mountain dwellers in the surroundings of Longzhou, a town in the Province of Guangxi, close to the North Vietnam border. Farther to the east, Lewis

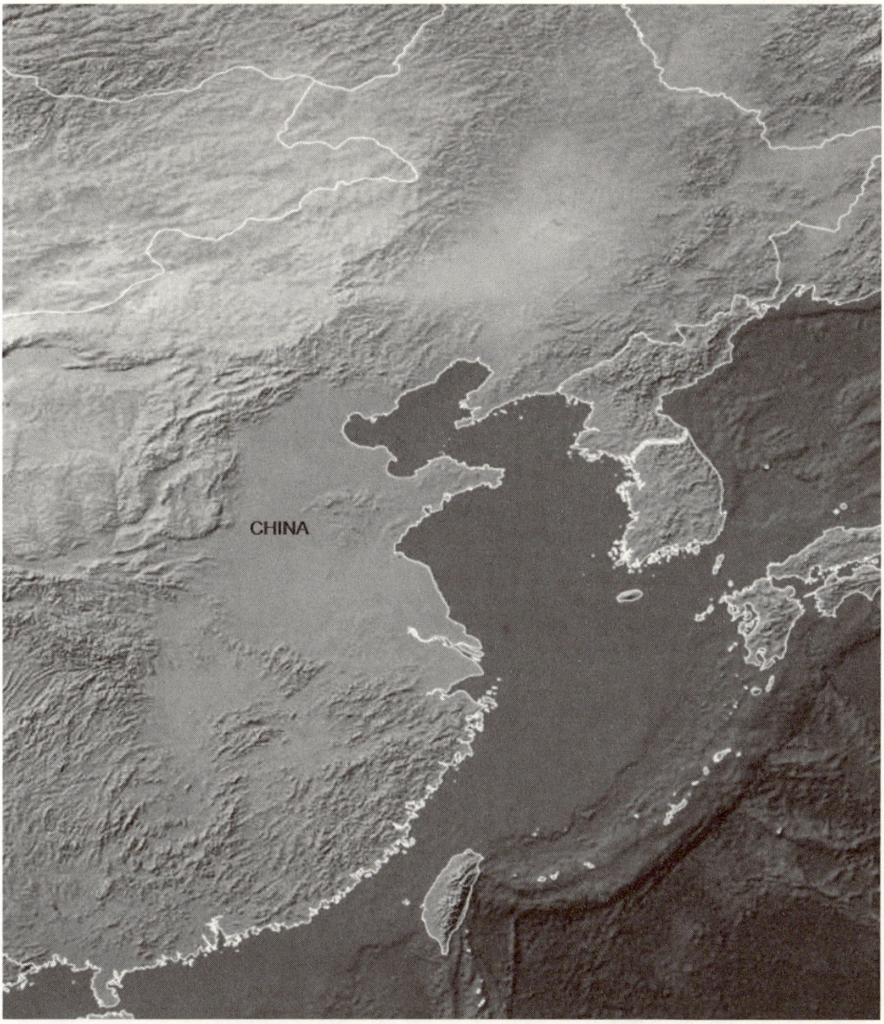

Figure 3.7 The topography of Eastern China.
Copyright: EUMETSAT

came upon a strong focus of goiter in the Province of Hunan, when journeying over the mountains between Lanshan and Lianzhou. Nearly at the top of the ridge was a village where he saw greatly enlarged thyroids in large numbers. The villagers told him that the disease was long-standing and that practically the entire adult population were victims.

Philippines

The Filipinos showed the highest frequency of goiter among people residing in the Orient. The disease seemed to be almost as prevalent in the Philippine Islands as in Switzerland.

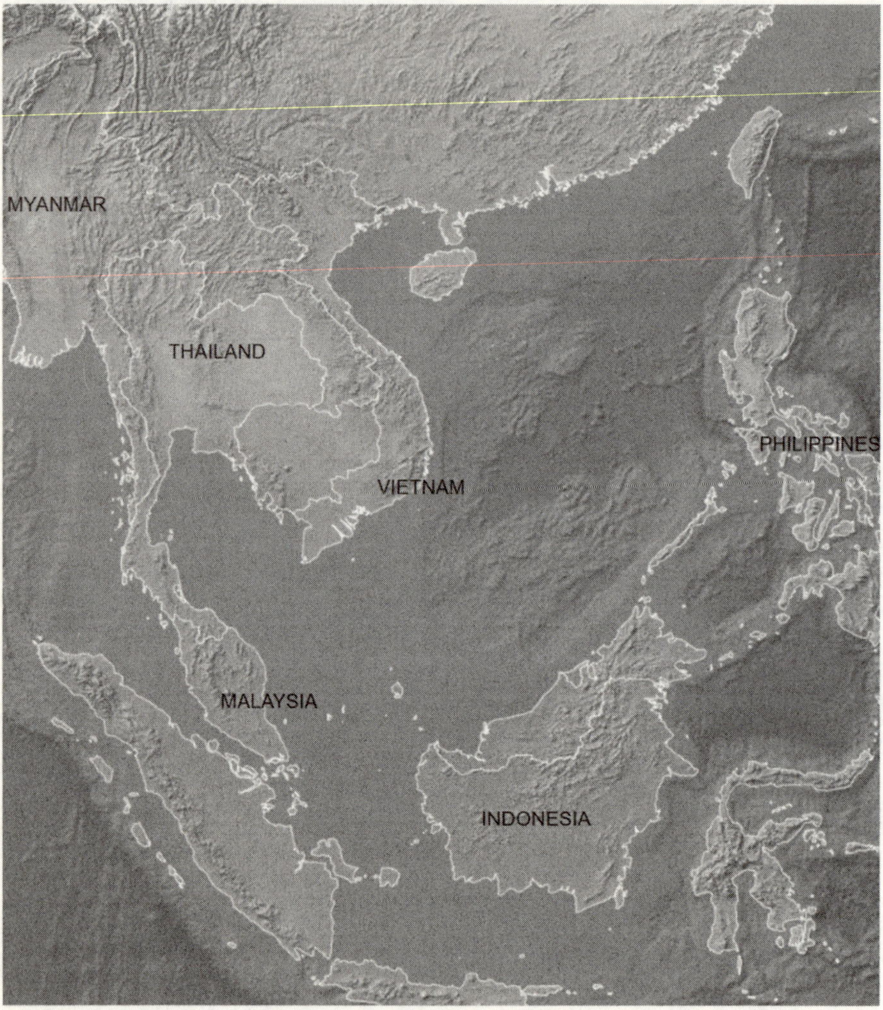

Figure 3.8 The topography of Southeast Asian countries—Myanmar, Thailand, Cambodia, Laos, Vietnam, Malaysia, Singapore, Indonesia, and Philippines. The population of these countries is approximately 680 million.

In summary, the geographical distribution of goiter and cretinism in various countries shows that there is a strong relationship between geography (mountains) and the severe forms of thyroid disease (goiter and cretinism).

References

1. Kelly FC, Snedden WW. Prevalence and geographical distribution of endemic goitre. In: *Endemic Goitre.* Monograph Series No. 44. Geneva: World Health Organization; 1960:27-234.
2. Clements FW, Moerloose JD, Desmet MP, et al. *Endemic Goitre.* Monograph Series No. 44. Geneva: World Health Organization; 1960.
3. Inglis J. *Treatise on English Bronchocele: with a Few Remarks on the Use of Iodine and Its Compounds.* London: Longman, Orme, Brown, Green, and Longmans; 1838:10.
4. Blackie GS. *Cretins and Cretinism,* A Prize Thesis of University of Edinburgh. Edinburgh: Maclachlan & Stewart and London: Simpkin, Marshall & Co.; 1855.
5. Koutras DA. Europe and the Middle East. In: Stanbury JB, Hetzel BS, eds. *Endemic Goiter and Endemic Cretinism.* John Wiley; 1980:83.
6. Yang Q, Zheng D. *Himalayan Mountain System;* 2004. In: Himalayas. https://en.wikipedia.org/wiki/Himalayas. Accessed May 8, 2022.
7. Stott H, Gupta SP. *Indian J. Med. Res.* 1934;21:649-655.
8. Stott H, Bhatia BB, Lal RS, Rai KC, *Indian J. Med. Res.* 1931;18:1059.
9. Geography of China. https://en.wikipedia.org/wiki/Geography_of_China. Accessed May 8, 2022.
10. Tai M, Tizhang L, Yubin T, Bingzhong C, Xianyi Z (Chu HL). The present status of endemic goitre and endemic cretinism in China.

In: *Food and Nutrition Bulletin*. The United Nations University Press; 1982:4(4).

11. China Administrative PRC. Wikipedia.org. https://commons.wikimedia.org/wiki/File:China_administrative_PRC.svg. Accessed May 8, 2022.

12. Heihe-Tengchong-Line. Wikimedia.org. https://commons.wikimedia.org/wiki/File:Heihe-tengchong-line.svg. Accessed May 8, 2022.

Chapter 4

The Cause of Thyroid Disease

As discussed in the previous chapter, the geography (mountains) provides us a clue to the cause of thyroid disease. Mountains were formed millions of years ago when tectonic plates, located below the earth's crust, collided against each other. Earth, with the continents and oceans, is made of seven major tectonic plates. For example, India is on a tectonic plate called Indian Plate, and China is on a tectonic plate called Eurasian Plate. When these plates collided millions of years ago, the Himalayan Mountains were formed along the boundary of India and China, i.e., along the boundary where the two plates collided.

Tectonic plates are composed of continental crust (earth layer) and ocean crust (oceans and the floor layer beneath them). When tectonic plates collided, what was once an ocean floor rose to top of the Earth in the form of mountains. Ocean floor is about 100 km (62 miles) thick and is made of shells, bones, and fossils of dead, sea animals from millions of years. This sea debris has now become limestone rocks in the mountains.

Mountains are primarily made of sedimentary rocks and metamorphic rocks. The two common types of sedimentary rocks are limestone and sandstone. In the context of thyroid disease, we are interested in limestone rocks.

i. Lemon, Lime, and Limestone

Before we go further, a brief clarification is required on the word *limestone.* Limestone is often confused with other similar sounding words, lemon, and lime.

Lemon is a fruit. It is yellow or green in color, sour in taste, and is used to make lemon juice or lemonade. Lime is also a fruit. It is the size of a tennis ball, green in color, with yellow spots when ripe. It is sweet in taste and is used to make lime juice. It is also called sweet lime.

Limestone is a rock. It is commonly called as chalk or lime (*not to be confused with lime fruit*). Limestone is formed from accumulated shells and corals in the sea over millions of years.

ii. Hard Water and Soft Water

A brief clarification is also required about the difference between hard water and soft water.

Water that has an excess of minerals like calcium and magnesium is called *hard water.* The excess minerals make the water *hard*, and hence the name hard water. Hard water is formed when water passes through limestone rocks under the earth's surface or on the surface of the earth. Water from limestone rocks or soil is usually hard. In our day-to-day use, hard water forms white flakes on utensils, faucets, and bathroom floors. Hard water does not produce much foam when we take bath with soap or body wash. We are interested in hard water in the context of thyroid disease. We will use the terms hard water and limestone-source water interchangeably in this book.

Water that does not have much quantity of minerals in it is called soft water. Rainwater is an example of soft water; there are little or no minerals in it. Soft water does not form flakes on utensils or on bathroom faucets and floors. Soft water produces good foam when we take bath with soap or body wash.

iii. John McClelland

In the previous chapter, we saw thyroid disease at a country level. In this chapter, we will see thyroid disease at a village level.

The findings detailed in this chapter are from the research of John McClelland, in India, between 1831 and 1835.[1] John McClelland was a British doctor who worked for the East India Company in India. His research is the finest ever done on thyroid disease. There were many researchers who did research on thyroid disease before and after him. But what sets him apart are his unique qualifications and his approach.

Although McClelland was a doctor by profession, he did significant work in geology. Geology is the study of rocks and earth. In 1836, he served as the Secretary of an organization that eventually became the Geological Survey of India, the premier geology survey body of India. Thus, McClelland had a unique combination of medical and geology skills. The best thyroid doctor in the world may not be able to find the cause of thyroid disease. Similarly, the best geologist in the world may not be able to find the cause of the thyroid disease. It was a combination of these skills that helped McClelland to find the cause of thyroid disease. Most other early researchers of thyroid disease were, by qualification, either doctors, chemists, medical researchers, travelers, architects, philosophers, or historians.

Another aspect which set McClelland apart from rest of the researchers was his approach. He studied thyroid disease independent of the prevailing theory about the cause. He merely collected data. He did not have any preconceived notion about the cause.

McClelland's research was primarily done in Kumaon, a district located in the Himalayan Mountain range in India. Kumaon is in the present-day Uttarakhand, a state in North India. The East India Company of Britain was ruling major parts of India at the time McClelland did his research. McClelland visited over 125 villages and surveyed 6,500 inhabitants for goiter and cretinism. He studied the rocks on which each village stood and the source of water of each village. Often, a particular village had more than one source of water. McClelland's approach was so thorough and meticulous that he studied the impact of each water source on the villagers. This was not an easy task to do in a foreign country about 200 years ago, in villages where people spoke in local languages.

In 1831, McClelland was posted as a medical in-charge of two military detachments at two different military posts in Kumaon. These two military posts were stationed at Lohaghat and Pithoragarh. McClelland's research was the result of residence in Kumaon while on regular duty with these regiments. The findings of his research in these two military posts are detailed on the following pages.

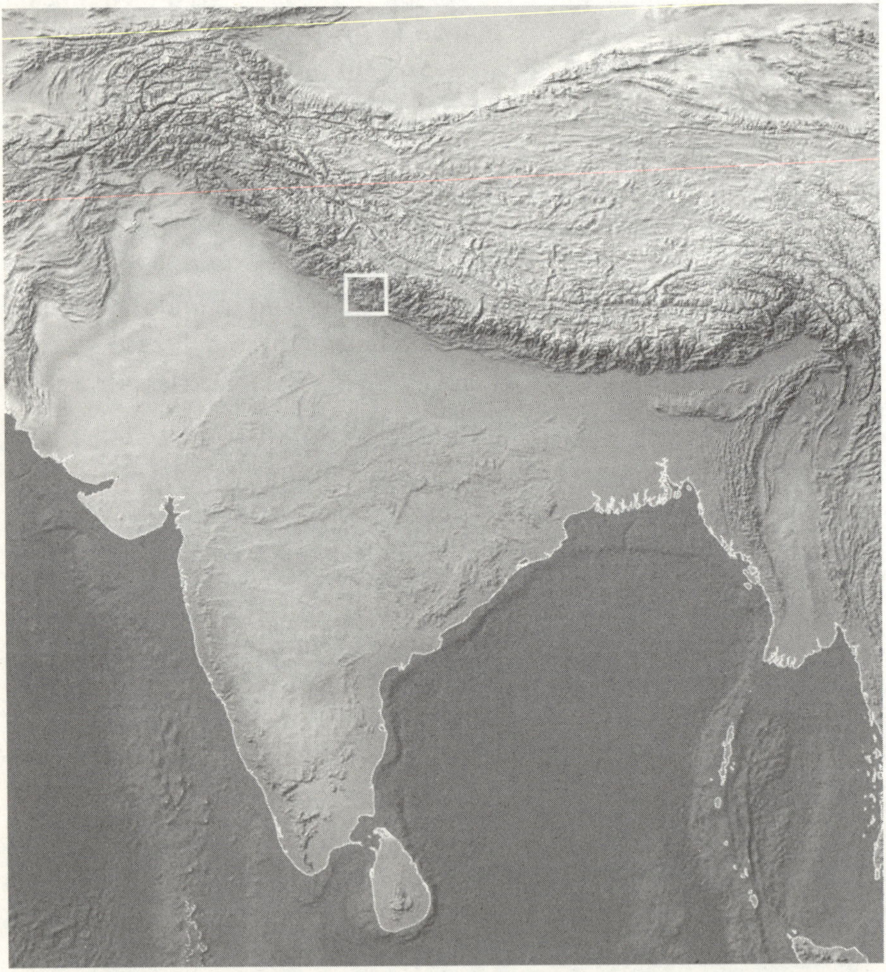

Figure 4.1 The square mark on the map shows the approximate location of Lohaghat, Pithoragarh, and the 126 villages discussed in this chapter.

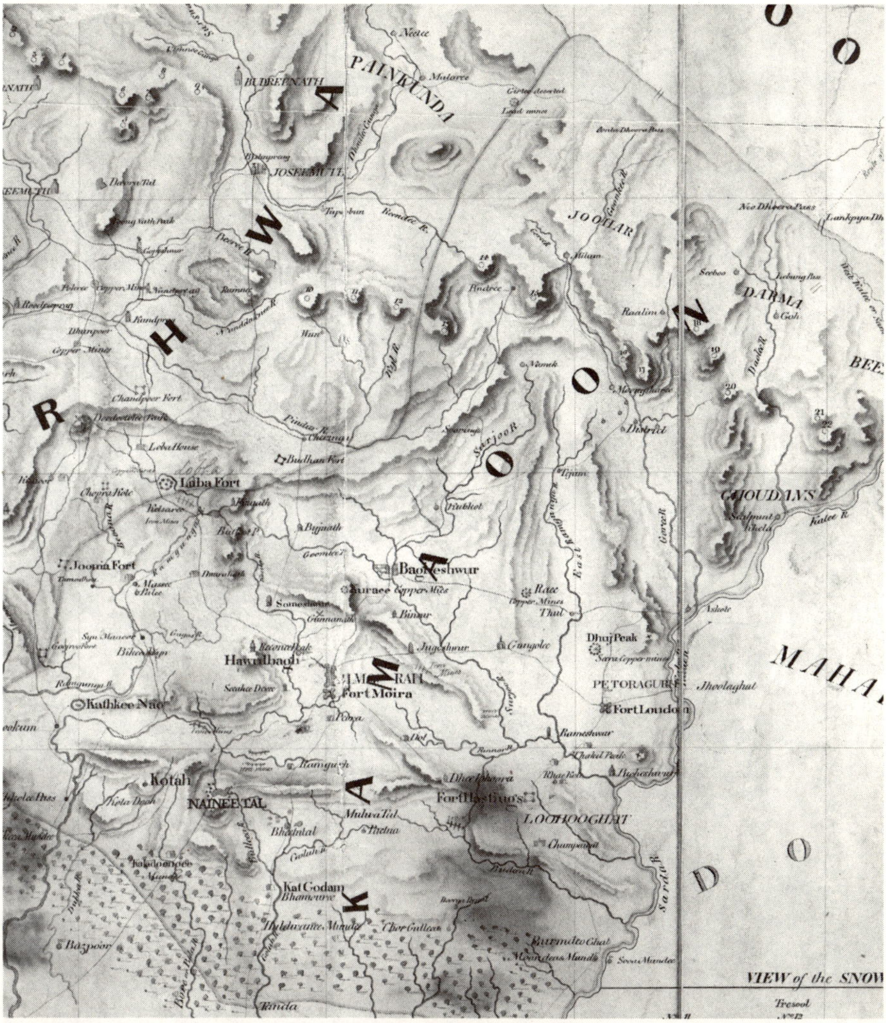

Figure 4.2 The 1846 map shows the location of Lohaghat and Pithoragarh at the foothills of the Himalayas. The map refers to old spellings of these places, Loohooghat and Petoragurh.

Image credit: Kumauni Archives

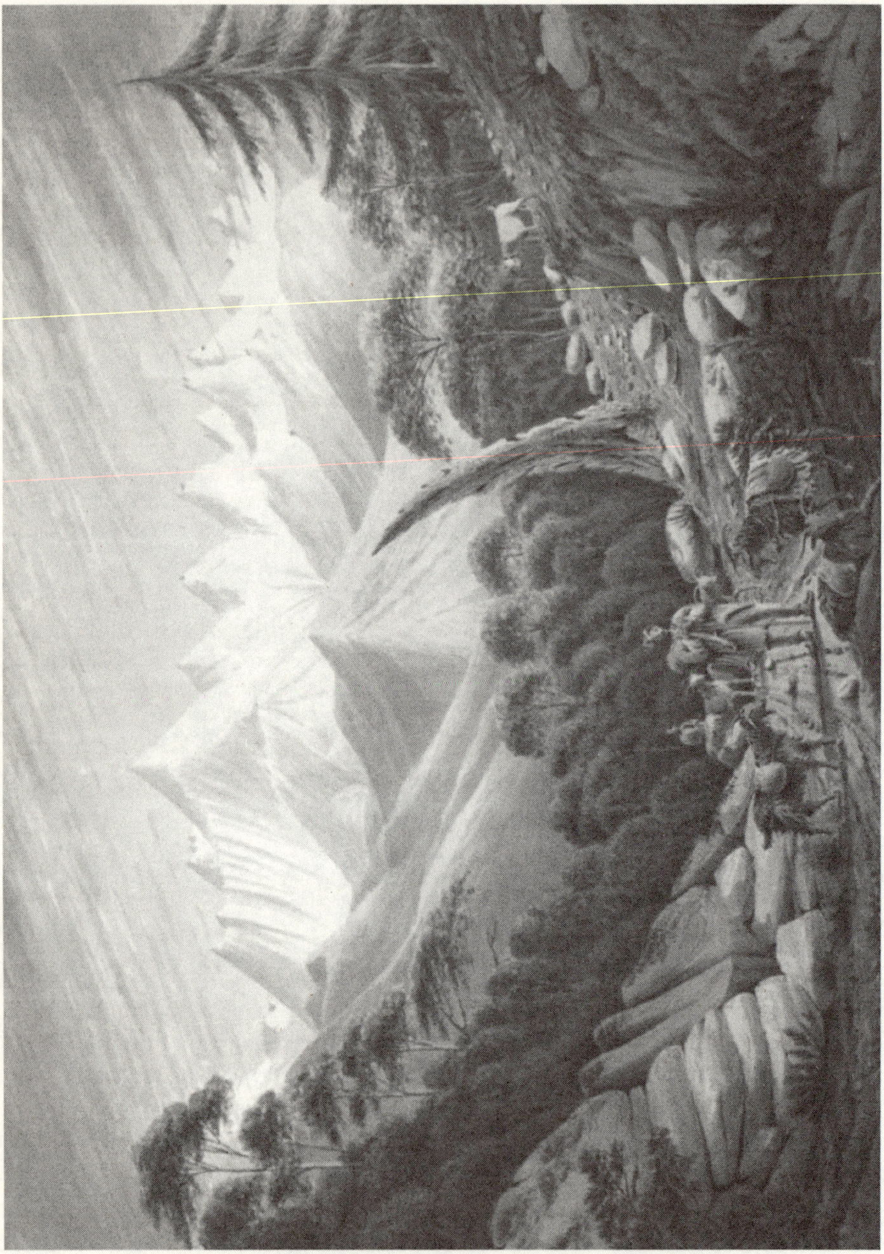

Figure 4.3 Water-colour painting showing the Himalayan Mountains from the Almora District, the neighboring district of Kumaon. Painting by James Manson (1791-1862), c.1826.

Image credit: Kumauni Archives

iv. Lohaghat

In 1831, Lohaghat was a small valley in Kumaon. It was half a mile wide and one and a half mile long in East West direction. The mean temperature was 60 °F (15 °C). The military cantonment was surrounded by hills that rose from 500 feet to 1000 feet above.

Clay-slate was the primary rock in this valley. There were other rocks, but their relative proportion was negligible. The water sources in the valley were the numerous springs that emerged from the clay-slate. The solid extracts in the water in this valley were not more than 1/13,000th part of the water.

In 1831, two companies of the 30th Native Infantry Regiment took possession of this post. After 3 years of residence at Lohaghat, not one soldier or the numerous camp followers, about 400 men, women, and children, were affected by goiter.

v. Pithoragarh

The cantonment of Pithoragarh was 15 miles in the north direction from Lohaghat. The cantonment was more open than Lohaghat. There were no higher elevations within the distance of 3–4 miles. The mean annual temperature at Pithoragarh was about 2 °F higher than Lohaghat.

The rocks in this vicinity were composed of clay-slate, however, extensive deposits of limestone supported these rocks.

Pithoragarh cantonment also had two companies of the 30th Native Infantry Regiment. Both Pithoragarh and Lohaghat had the same strength and the same number of camp followers. And both regiments entered the hills together.

Table 4.1 shows the number of goiter cases in each regiment.

Table 4.1 Number of goiter cases at Lohaghat and Pithoragarh

	Lohaghat	Pithoragarh
End of 1st year	0	0
End of 2nd year	0	5
End of 3rd year	0	15

We may note that Lohaghat had zero cases in three years. At Pithoragarh, however, about 4% of the regiment was affected by goiter at the end of three years.

In another context, McClelland mentions that goiter usually takes about six years to fully develop. Pithoragarh would have probably had an even higher number of goiter cases at the end of six years.

What's not mentioned in these findings is the number of moderate thyroid disease cases in each regiment. If the present-day testing methods were used, a significantly higher number of people would have probably been diagnosed with hypothyroidism at Pithoragarh. Mild cases may not have been easy to detect two hundred years ago.

McClelland made other observations at these two military posts. Table 4.2 provides a summary of the number of hospital admissions due to various diseases at both these two locations.

Table 4.2 Number of hospital admissions in Lohaghat and Pithoragarh from 1831 to 1834

Reason for hospital admission	Lohaghat	Pithoragarh
Fevers	167	232
Dysentery	7	88
Ulcers, chiefly of foot	44	56
Rheumatism	19	46
Slight injuries/wounds	2	21
Syphaloid diseases	7	14
Pulmonary afflictions	6	10
Diarrhea	32	5

We may note from Table 4.2 that almost every disease was higher at Pithoragarh than at Lohaghat. Dysentery cases were 10 times more in Pithoragarh than in Lohaghat (88 cases in Pithoragarh, 7 cases in Lohaghat). Dysentery is inflammation, especially in the colon. Diarrhea on the other hand is frequent passing of loose and watery stools. Pithoragarh, which had higher goiter cases also had higher intestinal inflammation cases. This shows a relationship between intestinal inflammation and thyroid disease.

Rheumatism cases were 150% more in Pithoragarh than in Lohaghat. Rheumatism is intermittent (on and off) pain affecting the joints or connective tissues. People with rheumatism usually have pains in knee joints, shoulder joints, finger joints, and other joints and connective tissues in the body. People suffering from thyroid disease often complain of rheumatic pains.

Fevers were 50% more in Pithoragarh than in Lohaghat. McClelland mentioned that the number of sick people admitted to the hospital at Pithoragarh was nearly twice that of admissions at Lohaghat.

From the above, we may conclude that the number of goiter cases and sick people were significantly higher in Pithoragarh than in Lohaghat. The two locations had similar weather and were located at similar altitude. The people in the cantonments were similar in all respects. Their dietary habits were similar. The only difference between the two places was the source of water. Lohaghat got its water from a clay-slate source, while Pithoragarh got its water from a mix of clay-slate and limestone source.

McClelland felt that he was favorably placed for conducting goiter research in comparison with any other researcher who may not have been exposed be to such contrasting locations in such a short distance. During the course of his study, McClelland noted that he was struck by the frequency of goiter in one portion of the district while another was exempt from the complaint—and this despite the similar circumstances in which the people lived in both these places. We are fortunate that McClelland did not restrict his study to the two military posts. He studied goiter disease in the villages surrounding these two military posts.

vi. Villages Near Lohaghat

McClelland studied goiter and cretinism in 43 villages near Lohaghat and the 3,700 inhabitants in them. Only 17 inhabitants in these villages were affected by goiter, which is less than 1% of the inhabitants. These villages near Lohaghat were located to the south of the Ramesa river. The geology of these villages and the goiter prevalence rate in these villages is detailed below.

Villages # 1 to 6 (Rykote, Patan, and four other villages)

These six villages were situated two miles north of Lohaghat at an altitude of 6,000 feet above the sea level. The mean annual temperature in these village was 60 °F. The villages were erected on iron-clay derived from disintegration of clay-slate. There were 200 inhabitants in these six villages, and none of them had goiter.

Villages # 7 to 15 (Nakote, Gourouly, Choka, Pimtolly, Jata, Borinkore, Neltokora, Chopota, and Seiligna)

These nine villages were situated on the northwest ascent of a mountain named Gomedace. The mean altitude of the villages was 4,300 feet and the mean temperature was 64 °F. These villages were erected on clay-slate. There were 800 inhabitants in these villages, and only four people with small goiter were noted among them.

Even these four people with goiter were aged. They informed McClelland that they acquired goiter in their youth while residing in a distant part of the country. We may note that people still had thyroid disease in old age, although they have moved away from the goiter-causing location in their youth. This shows that effects of goiter/thyroid disease are long-lasting. The neck swelling and other symptoms of goiter disease may not fully go away despite moving to a non-goiter area. But probably, these four people would have become more diseased if they had stayed back in the goiter village of their youth. Elsewhere, McClelland noted that people rarely lived beyond the age of 50 years in one of the worst goiter-affected villages.

Villages # 16 to 19

These four villages were located in the eastern descent of the Gomedace mountain in the valley of the Mahi Kalee River. The villages were erected on clay-slate. There were 150 inhabitants in these villages, and none of them had goiter.

Villages # 20 to 28 (Pansall, Cheemrouly, Konera, Leno Simela, Chomonnee, Lund, Katee, and Katully)

These villages were situated on low ridges and deep ravines. The villages were erected on primitive clay-slate. There were 800 inhabitants in these villages, and only three cases of goiter were found among them.

Villages # 29 to 37 (Agee, Nina, Choura, Ryem Deortola, Gorong, Sutura, Chakora, Wellishone)

These villages were erected on primitive clay-slate. There were 600 inhabitants, of whom only four were affected by goiter.

Villages # 38 to 45 (Bentally, Jarig, Babra, Goumana, Biouly, Guinora, Kakur, Barakote)

These villages were situated in deep valleys, on high ridges, and declivities. They were situated on slate and sandstone. There were 500 inhabitants in these villages, and six of them had goiter.

Villages # 46 to 52

These seven villages were four miles northwest of Lohaghat, near the Jeercoonee mountain. It was exceedingly rugged and for the most part inaccessible. Deep ravines enclosed it on three sides. On the south were the villages of Junera, Dostee, Thur, and Mura. Nothing can be more frightful than the localities of these villages, from the lofty cliffs and mountains which seem to overhang them, with deep chasms at angles of 30° below. They were erected on slate and sandstone. There were 400 inhabitants in these villages, and not a single case of goiter was recorded. We may note that despite the difficult terrain, there were no cases. Therefore, the terrain was not a cause of goiter.

Villages # 53 to 56 (Rigong, Chimtouly, Bursolly, and Popoulee)

The first two villages were surrounded by deep ravines and extensive forests. The last village was situated near the summit of a mountain, on hornblende slate. The first two villages were on low ridges of slate. There were 250 inhabitants in these villages, and none of them had goiter.

The first set of villages were in deep ravines and surrounded by forests. The air would be stuck in such places. The last village was on the summit of a mountain. There would be much freer movement of air. Yet, none of the villages had cases of goiter. This shows that confined or stuck air, which was often considered as a cause of goiter by researchers in Europe in the 19th century, was not the cause of goiter.

Table 4.3 provides a summary of goiter prevalence in the 43 villages that were located near the Lohaghat military post. The goiter prevalence in these 43 villages was about 0.5% (17 goiter cases out of 3,700 inhabitants).

Table 4.3 Summary findings in villages near Lohaghat

Village number	Rock-type on which the villages stood	Rock-type from which water was sourced	Total inhabi-tants	Goiter Cases
1–6	Clay-slate	Clay-slate	200	0
7–15	Slate	Slate	950	4
16–19	Clay-slate	Clay-slate	800	3
20–28	Clay-slate	Clay-slate	600	4
29–37	Clay-slate	Clay-slate	500	6
	Sandstone	Sandstone	200	0
46–52	Clay-slate	Clay-slate	200	0
	Hornblende-slate	Hornblende-slate	54	0
53–56	Slate	Slate	195	0
Total			**3,700**	**17**

vii. Villages Near Pithoragarh (in the Shore Valley)

The villages near the Pithoragarh military post had significantly higher rates of goiter than those in the villages near Lohaghat. This is similar to the difference in findings at the two military posts.

The villages near Pithoragarh were located across the Ramesa river in the Shore valley. In these villages, 12.5% of the population was affected by goiter. We may note the stark difference. On one side of Ramesa river, only 0.5% of the inhabitants are affected, and on the other side,

12.5% were affected. This was despite the fact that customs, religion, marriage practices, moral, and political ethos were similar in both these groups of villages. The details of the villages near Pithoragarh in the Shore valley are as below.

1. Beesty

The village was situated on the southern extremity of a low group of hills, in the center of Shore valley. It was built on clay-slate. It was supplied with water from the rocks in clay-slate. There were 60 inhabitants in this village. All of them were free from goiter, except for one elderly person, who had come years ago from another part of the neighborhood. The goiter in this elderly person had rather diminished after coming to reside in this village.

2. Pando

The village was half a mile north from the last described village. It was erected on clay-slate. But scattered blocks of limestone partly covered the surface of the slate, and a small bed of limestone terminated in a knoll, on which the village was erected. It was supplied with water from clay-slate. There were 25 inhabitants in the village. None of them had goiter.

The inhabitants of this village were Rajpoots, an upper caste. Caste is a social class segregation in Hinduism, the predominant religion in India. Since ancient times, different castes had different customs, eating habits, and marriage rituals. McClelland studied goiter incidence caste-wise to see if any peculiar habits of a caste could offer a clue to the cause of goiter.

3. Salmora

Salmora was the name given to a few huts situated at the northern extremity of the Shore valley. It was about a mile from the last described village. This village differed from the previous village in that it was erected on limestone. The village was supplied with water from limestone rocks. There were 14 inhabitants in this village, and six cases of goiter among them, i.e., 40% of the villagers had goiter. There was also one case of cretinism.

The inhabitants of this village were from two families of seven members each. One family were Rajpoots, and the other family were Doms, a lower caste. Among the Rajpoots, there were 2 cases of goiter and 1 case of cretinism. Among the Doms, there were 4 cases of goiter. The Rajpoot cretin was deaf and dumb, had a large head, and an idiotic expression.

4. Celouly

This was a small village, situated on the northern acclivity of the same knolls on which the first two villages in Shore valley were situated. It was erected on clay-slate and supplied with water from clay-slate. There were 25 inhabitants in the village. All of them were free from goiter. All of them belonged to Rajpoot caste.

5. Murh

This was a larger village than any of the previous villages in Shore valley and was situated close to the above village (Celouly), but at the base of an opposite mountain. It was erected on the junction of clay-slate and limestone. An extensive bed of granitine advanced close to the village. The granitine was mainly composed of limestone. The basins of the springs were situated in this rock, but the waters were most likely derived from the substratum, as the granitine in question was seldom observed to afford the springs. There were 70 inhabitants in the village. There were 5 cases of goiter, i.e., 7% of the villagers were affected by goiter. The village had an equal number of Rajpoots and Doms. Among Rajpoots, there were 2 cases of goiter, and among Doms, there were 3 cases of goiter.

6. Gooragong

This village was situated a mile northeast of Murh, about 200 feet above the Shore valley. It had an open aspect only on the southeast, and its temperature was consequently higher than those of the villages in the vicinity. The site of the village was alpine; more alpine than the seven villages at Jeercoonee (described in the previous section). That is, it was exceedingly rugged, and for the most part inaccessible, as deep ravines enclosed it. The village was built on coarse limestone. Lofty precipices of alpine limestone ascended abruptly behind it to a height of 2,000 feet. Water supply was from limestone rocks. There were 18 inhabitants in the village. There were 12 cases of enormous goiter, i.e., 66% of the villagers had goiter. Among the 10 Rajpoots, 7 had goiter (i.e., 70%), and among the 8 Doms, 5 had goiter (i.e., 63%).

7. Teebee

This village was situated three-fourth of a mile from the previous village. It was on an arm of the same mountain, which extended into the valley. It was 200 feet above the level of Shore valley. It was built on clay-slate, coated with an incrustation of limestone. It was watered by a stream which issued from the same source that supplied the above village. But in the present case, it was taken for use after running about a quarter of a mile in the natural channel. There were 20 inhabitants in the village. There were 7 cases of large goiter, i.e., 35% of the villagers were affected.

8. Stagalinge

This village was erected on an arm of a mountain, which extended the same distance into the valley as the previous village. The localities of both the villages were close, with similar aspects. It had the same elevation as the last village. It was erected on clay-slate rock and was supplied with water from a spring in clay-slate. This was the only aspect in which this village differed from the previous village. There were 40 inhabitants in this village, and there were only 2 cases of goiter; that is, only 5% of the villagers were diseased in comparison with the 35% in the previous village. Both these villages were similar in all aspects, except that this village got its water from clay-slate source and the previous village got its water from limestone source.

9. Panere

This was the name by which three small groups of houses were distinguished in the north-western extremity of the Shore valley. The elevation was 200 feet above the valley. Panere was built upon clay-slate. Two groups of houses used the water of a stream that descended a short way from its source in the limestone cap of the mountain above them.

There were 30 inhabitants in these two groups of houses. There were 4 cases of goiter. These two groups belonged to the Doms caste. The third group got its water from a spring in the clay-slate. There were 24 inhabitants in this group. All of them were free from goiter. The third group belonged to the Rajpoot caste.

10. Bajeetee

This village was situated on the southern ascent of a low ridge that intersected the valley from east to west. The village was built on clay-slate, coated with limestone matter. The villagers derived the water, which they used for culinary purposes, from two distinct wells sunk near the bed of a stream, which issued from the limestone cap of the adjoining mountain. The wells were so situated that they did not seem to be supplied by any independent spring, but rather from this stream, particularly during the dry season. There were 50 inhabitants in this village. There were 16 cases of goiter (i.e., 30%). The village had 20 Brahmins, an upper caste. Among them, there were 3 cases of goiter (i.e., 15%). The village had 30 Doms. Among them, there were 13 cases of goiter (i.e., 43%).

11. Popdeon

Popdeon was situated half a mile west of the previous village. There were no distinctions in the physical conditions in comparison to the last village. There were 80 inhabitants in the village and there were 18 cases of goiter (i.e., 20%) among them. There were 50 inhabitants of higher caste, and there were 8 cases of goiter among them (i.e., 15%). There were 30 inhabitants of lower caste, and there were 10 cases of goiter among them (i.e., 30%).

12. Panorah

Panorah was situated in the western extremity of Shore valley, about a mile west of the last village. The village was built on clay-slate, slightly coated with limestone matter. There were 90 inhabitants in this village, and there were 7 cases of goiter among them (i.e., 8%). But when we look at the goiter percentage by caste, the difference in prevalence of goiter is striking. There were 70 inhabitants of Brahmin caste. Of them, only 1 was affected by goiter (i.e., less than 2%). There were 20 inhabitants of Doms caste. Of them, 6 were affected by goiter (i.e., 20%). What explains such a huge difference? The Brahmins, the high caste inhabitants of this village, derived their water from a spring in clay-slate. As a prejudice, Hindus in ancient times denied the lower caste the privilege of drinking water from the same spring used by the upper caste. The excluded caste was forced, in this case as well as in many other cases in Kumaon, to use water from what they, as well as the Brahmins, believed to be impure sources. In this case, it was taken from a stream that issued from the same limestone caps that provided waters to the previous two villages.

13. Paruee

Paruee was lower down in the valley than any of the previous villages. It was about a quarter of a mile south of the same knoll on which Bajeetee (village no. 10 in Shore valley) was erected. The village was erected on clay-slate. It was surrounded by fine springs in the same rock. There were 60 inhabitants in this village, and all of them were free of goiter. All the inhabitants belonged to Brahmin caste.

14. Dungaunee

Dungaunee was situated half a mile south of the military cantonments, on the southern side of the low ridge, which intersected the valley from west to east. It was supplied with water from a spring in clay-slate. There were 25 inhabitants, and all of them were free from goiter.

15. Bagalla

Bagalla was situated a little lower in the valley than the last. It was erected on clay-slate. It was surrounded by springs in clay-slate. There were 40 inhabitants in this village, and none of them were affected by goiter. There were 18 inhabitants of higher caste and 22 inhabitants of lower caste.

16. Kumora

Kumora was situated a quarter of a mile east of Dungaunee. This village was elevated 50 feet above the Shore valley, on a small knoll forming part of the low ridge that intersected the valley. The ridge rose behind this and the following seven villages at a distance of 300 yards in their rear, to a height of 200 feet above them. This village and the following seven villages were situated on clay-slate. These villages were supplied with water from springs in the clay-slate. There were 70 inhabitants in this village, and there were no cases of goiter. The first three villages in the list were situated close to limestone, which formed in tabular masses in the rugged cap of the ridge. We may note that the mere presence of limestone in the villages was not causing goiter; only if water was supplied from a limestone source was it causing goiter. The seven villages below got their water from a clay-slate source.

17. (a) Jakane, 30 inhabitants, no case of goiter

18. (b) Chouser, 50 inhabitants, no case of goiter

19. (c) Beera, 40 inhabitants, no case of goiter

20. Boorikote, 100 inhabitants, no case of goiter

21. Kaseena, 15 inhabitants, no case of goiter

22. Kosooly, 25 inhabitants, no case of goiter

23. Lailure, 100 inhabitants, no case of goiter

In all the above villages described so far, there is an interesting trend. These villages, which did not have cases of goiter, were those which were in a line along the base of the central ridge of the Shore valley, beginning with Paruree (village # 13) and extending eastward to Lailure (village # 23).

Now, let us see villages that were affected by goiter.

24. Murakote

On each side of this village were other villages that were affected. They consisted of two groups. One, a mile distant in the southeast portion of the valley. The other, a mile distant in the opposite direction. Both these groups were disposed in lines parallel to the line of healthy villages. The locality of the following villages in the southeast portion of the valley had a striking resemblance in the external appearance and geological structure to the villages marked a, b, c (i.e., village # 17, 18, 19), whose inhabitants were insulated from the limestone strata, as they derived water from springs in the clay-slate.

25. (d) Kutkora, 15 inhabitants, 5 goiters (i.e., 30%)

26. (e) Baldakote, 14 inhabitant, 7 goiters (i.e., 50%)

27. (f) Batuda, 16 inhabitants, 10 goiters (i.e., 60%)

The above three villages constituted the southwestern line. These villages were erected on a conglomerate of limestone, with fragments of clay-slate, and partly on clay-slate coated with limestone. A clay-slate mountain supporting a massive cap of limestone ascended to an altitude of 300 feet above them, pouring out numerous fountains, from which the immense beds of limestone on which these villages stood were derived. The peculiarity of the rocks from which the waters were derived was the only way in which the inhabitants of these villages marked d, e, f, differed from those of a, b, c. The altitude, aspect, temperature, religion, and morals of the inhabitants of both groups of villages were the same.

The villages below were located on the northeast extremity of the Shore valley.

28. Deota

Deota was a long village that occupied half a mile at the foot of Durge mountain. The village was situated about 100 feet above the level of the valley. It was chiefly composed of limestone. The village was built on a conglomerated rock, composed of limestone, inclosing mosses and fragments of other rocks. There was a spring situated in the valley, at about hundred yards from the village. The water burst forth with strong ebullition from numerous veins, in quantities of 40 gallons a minute. The water gave adhesive properties to the sand and gravel by which it was surrounded. The ancestors of inhabitants of this village, perhaps aware of the noxious effects of the spring, had an aqueduct formed. The aqueduct supplied water from a distant source into the Brahmin portion of the village. The aqueduct was reserved exclusively for Brahmins. But during the rainy season, when water was plentiful, the Rajpoots also used the water of the aqueduct. But the Doms had no alternative at any season, but to use water from the limestone spring. The impact of different sources of water on people of different castes was as below.

Brahmins—There were 20 inhabitants. All of them were free from goiter.

Rajpoots—There were 40 inhabitants. There were 26 cases of goiter among them (i.e., 66% were affected).

Doms—There were 40 inhabitants. All of them were affected by goiter (i.e., 100%).

To what cause can we ascribe the immunity of one caste of inhabitants of this village and the almost universal affection of the other two castes? People of all the three castes were well fed. They did not have to work hard as their land produced the requisites of life without much labor. Difference of caste did not imply a difference in monetary circumstances and consequently comforts of life. The observations in this village alone are sufficient to show that water from limestone source is the cause of goiter.

29. Ninee

Ninee was also situated at the foot of Durge mountain, within a mile of the last described village. The village was partly on clay-slate. The village was partly detached from the base of the mountain by a small ravine, only a few yards wide; that is, this village was detached by only a few yards from the problematic goiter-producing waters of the mountain. The village was supplied by a small but sufficient spring in the clay-slate. There were 80 inhabitants in the village, and none of them had goiter. The inhabitants belonged to the Rajpoot caste.

30. Chonda

Chonda was also located at the foot of Durge mountain, about two miles east of Deota. The village was built on a conglomerate of limestone, inclosing fragments of slate and limestone. The inhabitants used the water of a stream, which descended from the acclivity of the mountain, depositing limestone. There were 25 inhabitants in the village, and 7 of them had goiter (i.e., 30%). For convenience, a few years ago, a portion of the stream was conducted via an artificial channel, through the cultivable land, to the village. There was reason to believe that this had modified the virulence of the water, as the goiters of those affected did not increase, as they used to do.

31. Sunn

Sunn was a small village about a mile east of the previous village. This village was also watered by a stream that descended from the mountain acclivity made of limestone. There was one family of Brahmins with 10 members, and 5 of them had goiter (i.e., 50% were affected).

32. Oliel and Cubulcola

Oliel and Cubulcola were two small hamlets, situated 3 miles eastward of the previous village in the direction of the strata. These two villages were situated in the most pleasing amphitheater, completely sheltered from the northerly and westerly winds, and partly also from those of the south. The villages were exposed to the full power of the sun, until a few hours before it set. These villages were chiefly composed of limestone. There were 25 inhabitants in these villages, 13 had goiter, and 10 were cretins. Of the cretins, a whole family was deaf and dumb. They were also deficient in sight. They did not show any reactions to the passions of joy or fear.

33. Bagultolly

Bagultolly was two miles east of the last described village. It was about 1,500 feet below the level of Shore valley, in what may be called the valley of the Mahi Kalee. Its aspect and locality were confined by mountains, which from this low situation seem to be of great height. It was built on clay-slate and partly watered by a spring in that rock and partly by a stream from the mountain. There were 25 inhabitants in the village, and 4 of them had goiter.

34. Bescolly

Bescolly was nearly on the same level as the previous village. But instead of being an enclosed valley, it was situated on an exposed low ridge. It was composed of clay-slate but covered by the usual calcareous conglomerate. It was watered by fountains that poured from the mountain acclivities. These mountain acclivities were composed of limestone. There were 25 inhabitants in the village, of them 10 were affected by goiter i.e., 40% of the villagers were affected.

35. Gooraght

Gooraght was situated two miles northeast of the previous village. It was built partly on clay-slate and partly on the conglomerate that contained, in addition to the usual rocks, blocks of common serpentine. Water was supplied from the mountain acclivity. There were 24 inhabitants in the village. Of them, 10 had goiter, i.e., 40% of the villagers were affected. A father and two sons were cretins. The sons were both deaf and dumb.

36. Chupuckea, 40 inhabitants, no goiter

37. Suakote, 40 inhabitants, no goiter

38. Murakote, 40 inhabitants, no goiter

The above three villages were in continuation of the line of villages that were exempt from goiter. These three villages were erected on clay-slate. Some blocks of overlying limestone were strewn about the neighborhood of these villages. But clay-slate sources provided plentiful supply of water for use.

39. Kotilla and Ruena

In the lowest part of the watershed of Shore valley, where the different streams collected their waters into a river, there was a partial sandstone formation, on which the following two villages were erected: (a) Kotilla, 50 inhabitants, with no goiter, and (b) Ruena, 50 inhabitants, with no goiter.

40. Deorcolla and Dingas

These villages were situated lower down the valley of the small river just mentioned above. They were surrounded by many of the highest mountains in Kumaon. These villages were erected partly on a magnesian limestone and partly on clay-slate. The surrounding acclivities were overspread with overlying masses of limestone. There were 40 inhabitants in the two villages, and none of them were affected by goiter.

Table 4.4 provides a summary of villages near Pithoragarh (in the Shore valley).

Table 4.4 Summary findings in villages near Pithoragarh (Shore valley)

Village number	Rocks on which the village was erected	Rocks from which the water was derived for use of inhabitants	Total inhabi-tants	Goiter cases	Goiter cases (in %)
1	Clay-slate	Clay-slate	60	–	–
2	Clay-slate	Clay-slate	25	–	–
3	Transition limestone	Limestone	14	6	40%
4	Clay-slate	Clay-slate	25	–	–
5	Granatine and clay-slate	Granatine	70	5	7%
6	Conglomerate of limestone, slate and limestone	Limestone	18	12	60%
7	Clay-slate coated with limestone	Limestone	20	7	35%
8	Clay-slate	Clay-slate	40	2	5%
9	Clay-slate	Limestone and slate	54	4	7%
10	Clay-slate incrusted with limestone	Limestone	50	16	30%
11	Clay-slate incrusted with limestone	Limestone	80	18	20%

Village number	Rocks on which the village was erected	Rocks from which the water was derived for use of inhabitants	Total inhabi-tants	Goiter cases	Goiter cases (in %)
12	Clay-slate	Limestone and slate	90	7	8%
13	Clay-slate	Clay-slate	60	–	–
14	Clay-slate	Clay-slate	25	–	–
15	Clay-slate	Clay-slate	40	–	–
16	Clay-slate	Clay-slate	70	2	3%
17	Clay-slate	Clay-slate	30	–	–
18	Clay-slate	Clay-slate	50	–	–
19	Clay-slate	Clay-slate	40	–	–
20	Clay-slate	Clay-slate	100	–	–
21	Clay-slate	Clay-slate	15	–	–
22	Clay-slate	Clay-slate	25	–	–
23	Clay-slate	Clay-slate	100	–	–
24	No data	No data	–	–	–
25	Clay-slate coated with limestone	Limestone	15	5	30%
26	Clay-slate coated with limestone	Limestone	14	7	50%
27	Conglomerate of limestone, slate and limestone	Limestone	16	10	60%
28	Conglomerate of limestone and fragments of slate	Limestone	100	60	60%
29	Clay-slate	Clay-slate	80	-	-
30	Conglomerate of limestone and fragments of slate	Limestone	25	7	30%
31	Clay-slate	Limestone	10	5	50%
32	Clay-slate and limestone	Limestone	25	13	50%
33	Clay-slate and limestone	Limestone	25	4	15%

Village number	Rocks on which the village was erected	Rocks from which the water was derived for use of inhabitants	Total inhabi-tants	Goiter cases	Goiter cases (in %)
34	Clay-slate and limestone	Limestone	25	10	40%
35	Conglomerate of limestone, slate and serpentine	Limestone	24	10	40%
36	Clay-slate and scattered blocks of limestone	Clay-slate	40	–	–
37	Clay-slate and scattered blocks of limestone	Clay-slate	40	–	–
38	Clay-slate	Clay-slate	40	–	–
39	Partial sandstone formation	Partial sandstone	100	–	–
40	Clay-slate and magnesium limestone	Clay-slate	40	–	–
	Total		**1,720**	**210**	**12%**

Table 4.4 clearly shows that drinking water originating from limestone strata/rocks causes goiter. The villages with the highest percentage of goiter cases got their water from limestone rocks. Drinking water originating from clay-slate sources did not cause goiter.

viii. Findings in a few other valleys near Shore Valley

Findings in many other villages in valleys near Shore valley further confirm that drinking water originating from limestone strata/rocks is the cause of goiter.

41. Valley of the Ramgungah river

There were eight villages in this valley, Busar, Kuttygang, Tulsar, Sangur, Domera, Chumalloo, and two others. These villages were situated 8 miles west of Shore valley. The valley was about 1,800 feet above the sea level. The lowest village was 400 feet above the bed of the river. The mountain acclivities on each side ascended at angles of about 20° to a height of 3,000 or 4,000 feet. The direction of the valley was from north to south. The direction of strata was from southeast to northwest. The limestone formations consequently crossed the valley obliquely. The villages were interspersed throughout the valley, at different altitudes. All the villages were erected on limestone.

There were 100 inhabitants in these villages, and 60 of them were affected by goiter (i.e., 60% were affected). The inhabitants of these villages were Rajpoots.

42. Valley of Kalapany

The valley of Kalapany adjoined the northern extremity of Shore valley. It extended 6 to 8 miles to the west, where it descended into the valley of the Ramgungah. It was probably one of the lowest inhabited places in Kumaon. It was closely surrounded by mountains, some of which ascended 6,000 feet above the river, at angles subtending from 20° to 30°. This valley contained a few villages. The presence or absence of goiter was marked by the same circumstances that were observed in the Shore valley.

The following two villages were most remarkable in the contrast they presented with respect to goiter.

a) Beechelly

This village was situated in the lowest part of the valley. It was surrounded by mountains of transition limestone and was erected on an alluvial deposit. The alluvial deposits were formed from the debris of other rocks and cemented loosely with calcareous matter. There were 70 inhabitants in the village, and there were 30 cases of goiter among them. There were 50 Rajpoots and 20 Doms in the village.

b) Reunna

This village was situated a mile to the east of the previous village. This village was as much surrounded by mountains as the last village and was only 50 feet higher. It was erected on the side of a knoll of a transition slate. The village had no springs. Hence, the inhabitants used the water of the river which flowed from the valley of Barabice (next village). There were 50 inhabitants in the village, only one of them had goiter. The inhabitants of this village were Rajpoots.

43. Valley of Barabice

The valley of Barabice was situated 12 miles north from the Shore valley, at an elevation of 4,000 feet. It was somewhat of an oval shape, extending 4 miles from east to west, and 2 miles from north to south. The eastern extremity of the valley was composed of clay-slate containing beds of talc. There were 5 villages in this end of the valley, with 152 inhabitants. But only 1 case of goiter was recorded among them.

The western extremity of the valley was bounded by a low ridge, which was formed from limestone. These rocks rested on clay-slate. In this end of the valley, there were 6 villages with 192 inhabitants. Of them, 70 were affected by goiter disease. But these 70 people were not equally distributed among these villages. The following two instances illustrate the diversity that prevailed in this aspect.

a) Ager

The villagers used water that flowed from an old copper mine, which was situated in limestone. There were 50 inhabitants in this village. Of them, 40 had large goiters i.e., 80% were affected. There were 20 inhabitants who were cretins. A few of the cretins had goiters too.

c) Ducygong

It was situated half a mile from the previous village, Ager. It was situated on the same rock as Ager. The villagers used water of a spring in clay-slate. There were 50 inhabitants in this village. None of the inhabitants were affected by goiter or cretinism. The villagers belonged to Brahmin and Rajpoot castes.

The incidence of goiter and cretinism in these two villages is another classic example to show that limestone-source water is the cause of thyroid disease.

44. Valley of Deodara

It was situated on the southern side of the Shore valley. It was divided from the Shore valley by a detached mountain of clay-slate, with a slight deposit of tubular limestone on its summit. The opposite side of the valley was bounded by Takill, a very loft mountain. This valley contained two large villages and several smaller ones. It was well watered by numerous springs in clay-slate. There were 250 inhabitants in this valley. Only 4 of them were affected by goiter (i.e., 2%). Even these 4 people were confined to a small village, which had 20 inhabitants. This small village was immediately beneath the limestone cap of the mountain, which divided the valley from Shore valley.

45. Valley of Goran

It was situated on the western side of the Shore valley. This valley was composed of a variety of rocks. But the villages were generally erected on clay-slate, which abounded in springs of pure water. The valley had 7 villages with 179 inhabitants. There were 16 cases of goiter among the villagers, i.e., 9% were affected. Of these 16 cases, 9 belonged to a small village of 24 inhabitants called Majara. The inhabitants of this village derived their water from a stream which rose from the limestone of the Oudepore mountains on the south side of the valley.

46. Valley of Roilputty

The valley of Roliputty was about 7 miles distant from the valley of Shore valley. It extended along the southwest foot of Takill. It was extremely wild and alpine. The valley had only 2 villages.

a) Tomilly

The village was situated on a transition slate, which contained no water. Consequently, water was procured form a stream that flowed in a small cascade over the rocky precipices of limestone. There were 25 inhabitants in the village, of whom, 6 (24%) had goiters and 8 (i.e., 30%) were cretins.

b) Kurkolly

The village was situated on the same rock as the first, but at a lower and more distant portion of the valley. It was furnished with water from the same rivulet, after it had run about a mile and half along the valley. There were 25 inhabitants in the village. But only 1 of them was affected by goiter.

47. Valley of Beechar

This valley was connected with the southwestern extremity of the Shore valley. It was divided from it only by a low, narrow ridge. The watershed of the valley descended from the northwest and was composed of clay-slate. On this was a village of 40 inhabitants. All were free from goiter.

On the lower side of the valley, and near the base of a lofty mountain, were two villages situated on a knoll of argillaceous slate, whose surface was coated with a slight calcareous/limestone incrustation. One village had 20 inhabitants, who were Brahmins. Of them, 5 were affected by goiter disease (i.e., 25%). The second village had 20 inhabitants, who were Doms. Of them, 10 were affected by goiter disease (i.e., 50%). Some of the goiter tumors were extremely large, even in children of 10 years age. Water in these villages was from two springs situated close to each other. The springs resembled the spring at Deota (village # 28). The source of the water in the springs was from veins situated between limestone and clay-slate rocks. Table 4.5 summarizes the findings in the villages in valleys near Shore valley.

Table 4.5 Summary findings in villages in valleys near Shore valley

Village number	Name of the valley	Rocks on which the village was erected	Rocks from which the water was derived for use of inhabitants	Total inhabi-tants	Goiter cases	Goiter cases (in %)
41	Valley of Ramgungah river	Limestone	Limestone	100	60	60%
42	Valley of Kalapany (1) Beechelly	Conglomerate of limestone	Limestone	70	30	40%

Village number	Name of the valley	Rocks on which the village was erected	Rocks from which the water was derived for use of inhabitants	Total inhabi-tants	Goiter cases	Goiter cases (in %)
	(2) Reunna	Transition slate	River	50	1	2%
43	Valley of Barabice (1) Eastern extremity	Clay-slate	Clay-slate	152	–	–
	(2) Western extremity	Limestone	Limestone	192	70	35%
44	Valley of Deodars (1)	Clay-slate	Clay-slate	225	–	–
	(2)	Clay-slate	Limestone	25	4	16%
45	Valley of Goron (1)	Limestone	Limestone	24	9	35%
	(2)	Clay-slate	Clay-slate	125	5	4%
	(3)	Granatine	Granatine	30	2	7%
46	Valley of Roilputty (1) Tomilly	Clay-slate	Limestone	25	6	25%
	(2) Kurkolly	Clay-slate	Limestone (after 1.5-mile runoff)	25	1	4%
47	Valley of Beechar, first village	Clay-slate	Clay-slate	20	–	–
	Valley of Beechar, second village	Clay-slate, incrusted with limestone	Limestone	20	15	75%
Total				**1,123**	**203**	**18%**

The Connection Between Goiter and Cretinism

There was not one cretin in any of the villages that were exempt from goiter. As noted earlier, McClelland found that when goiter prevailed to the extent of more than 50% in a population, there were 30% cretins, and when goiter did not extend above 9%, there were no cretins. In the village Goseragong, for example, the people were generally affected by goiter, yet there were no cretins among them. The same may be said of Deota. But in the villages of Salmora, Oliel, Gooraght, Tomilly and Ager, which had 138 inhabitants, 76 had goiter and 42 were cretins.

ix. Summary of McClelland's Research

A space upwards of 1,000 square miles was the subject of research by John McClelland. From Tables 4.6 and 4.7, we can see that goiter and cretinism, the relatively severe forms of thyroid disease, were primarily caused by drinking water from a limestone water source.

Table 4.6 Summary of McClelland's Research (absolute numbers)

Source of water (Strata/rocks)	Number of villages	Number of inhabitants	Number of goiter cases	Number of cretinism cases
Limestone	35	1,160	390	34
Clay-slate	71	3,957	29	0
Granatine	2	100	7	0
Hornblende-slate and mica-slate	1	50	0	0
Steatitic Sandstone	3	200	0	0
Partial sandstone	1	40	0	0
Granite and Genesis	0	0	0	0
Total	**126**	**6,543**	**436**	**34**

Table 4.7 Summary of McClelland's Research (percentage and proportion)

Source of water (Strata/ rocks)	Goiter		Cretinism	
	Inhab- itants affected by goiter	Proportion of inhabi- tants affect- ed by goiter	Inhab- itants affected by cretinism	Propor- tion of inhabitants affected by cretinism
Limestone	33.3%	1 in 3	8.25%	1 in 12
Clay-slate	0.7%	1 in 135	0	0
Granite	0.2%	1 in 500	0	0
Genesis	0.2%	1 in 500	0	0
Sandstone	0	0	0	0
Hornblende- slate	0	0	0	0
Mica-slate	0	0	0	0

x. Limestone-Source Water/Hard Water Linked to Thyroid Disease in Other Countries Too

India was not the only country where limestone source water and hard water were implicated as the cause of thyroid disease. Hard water was identified as the primary cause of goiter and cretinism in other geographies too.

Europe—Limestone is the Predominant Rock in the Alps Mountain Range

If we examine the geological structure of the affected countries in the Alps, we find that they all abundantly contain lime.

The following observations in Europe were made by George Blackie in 1855 in his *Cretins and Cretinism*, a Prize thesis of the University of Edinburgh.[2]

A bed of limestone and magnesian limestone occupies a great portion of the Alps region in Austria and Switzerland. The limestone belt covers

Tyrol (a state in west Austria), the whole of Grisons (a canton in east Switzerland), the Cantons of Schwytz, Uri, Obwalden and Nidwalden (in Switzerland), the greater part of the shores of the Lake Lucerne, then passing southwest, including Brienz, with its lake, and that of Thun, the Swiss mountains Faulhorn, Scheideck and Stockhorn, the Swiss passes of Gemmi and Zweizimmen, the Swiss towns of Loeche, Sierre and Sion, Mount Jaman, and Vevay, where it reaches the Lake of Geneva, along which it courses, stretching nearly as far south as Chamonix (a resort area near the junction of France, Switzerland, and Italy, located at the base of Mont Blanc, the highest summit in the Alps) and including Cluses and Bonneville (in France).

Another great belt of limestone covers the Rhône River from Brieg, as far as Furca in one direction, and Airolo and the Pass of Splügen in another. In support of the lime water theory, this was precisely that district in Switzerland and its adjoining territories where goiter and cretinism most abounded. It is another impressive fact that in the two beds of granite and gneiss, which interrupted the great limestone field, namely, the Bernese Oberland and the Mt. St. Gothard, goiters were rare, and cretinism probably did not exist.

In Swiss areas such as Martigny, Andermatt, and Geneva, the first two of which stood on granite, and none on limestone, were also liable to goiter. In Martigny, people suffered from goiter to a great amount. But there was an explanation for this. The inhabitants of Martigny drank the lime-impregnated water of the Rhône River, which had in all its course followed the lime district, with the exception in this city. Andermatt was supplied by Reuss river, rushing down from the Fucra and from a stream running from the Lake of Lucandro, near the summit of the Gothard. The people of Geneva were supplied with lime in the water of their lake.

The great limestone rocks at Cluse in Savoy formed one of the most striking features in the landscape; and between Balme and Maglan, in the same neighborhood, there were many cretins.

Dr. Mottard mentioned the case of a so-called goiter well, near St. Julien in Maurienne, France, the water of which was *saturated with lime*, and the use of which produced goiter in a couple of months. He mentioned that five young men voluntarily drank its water and developed goiter in order to be free from military service.

England

In 1838, in England, Dr. James Inglis, a physician and Member of The Royal College of Surgeons, UK, noted that presence of magnesian limestone always predicted the coexistence of goiter.[3(p23)] He noted that there was a ridge of magnesian limestone running from North to South through the center of Yorkshire, and margining the shires of Derby and Nottingham. All along this line, there was goiter to a great extent, whereas on diverging to either side of this line, goiter was found to diminish. The towns situated on this ridge were Nottingham, Alfreton, Chesterfield, Rotherham, Ackworth, Pontefract, Abberford, Wetherby, Knaresborough, Boroughbridge, and Ripon. After this the magnesian limestone dipped, and then reappeared in the county of Durham. It continued its course almost due north from Darlington to South Shields, where at Tynemouth it met the sea. In many of these towns Dr. Inglis noted goiter.

Between 1923 and 1930, Dr. P. H. J. Turton conducted detailed investigations on the distribution of goiter in Derbyshire.[4] He examined 40,000 students between ages 8 and 13 attending Derbyshire elementary schools and found that goiter rates varied according to age. The goiter rate was between 1% and 10% for girls and 0.5% and 4% for boys. The whole of Derbyshire was situated on mountain limestone, and areas with carboniferous limestone were always goitrous; and when a number of places were supplied with water from sandstone, the goiters greatly diminished or disappeared. The incidence of goiter in limestone areas as compared to sandstone areas was 4:1.

In the vicinity of Lyne, in Peeblesshire, Scotland, in the limestone rock areas, cases of goiter were frequent, and the same pattern was noted in other parts of the country.[2]

Canada

Dr. Richardson, the fellow traveler of Franklin who traveled to the North Pole, observed that the disease attacked only those who drank water of the Saskatchewan River, the water of which was hard. Dr. Richardson, in his account of goiter in Edmonton, Canada, remarked that the soil was calcareous (rich in *lime*), and contained many *fragments of limestone.*[3(p13)]

China

In Northeast China, studies indicated that the highest rates of goiter were in areas underlain by pre-Cambrian and *limestone formations.*[5(p179)]

In West China, the patchy distribution of goiter was explained on geological grounds.[5(p176)] In the western part of the Yunnan province, before the canyons of the Mekong and Salween, the country was composed of irregular ranges of upper grasslands and undulating plains, where pastoral agriculture was intensively practiced. Much of this country was on *porous limestone soil*, and it was here, in remote villages, that goiter was evident both in man and his flocks and herds.[5(p176)]

Colombia

In 1808, Francisco Jose de Caldas, a noted Colombian naturalist and patriot, repeatedly mentioned goiter in his writings. Apparently, he was the first in Colombia to attribute the disease to the quality of the local drinking waters, *some excessively charged with lime* and others with calcium sulfate, iron, and decaying vegetation.[5(p41)]

In summary, the observations in various countries further confirm that water from limestone source is the primary cause of goiter and cretinism, the severe forms of thyroid disease.

References

1. McClelland J. An inquiry into the nature and causes of goitre. In: *Some Inquiries in The Province of Kemaon, Relative to Geology, and Other Branches of Natural Science.* Calcutta: Thacker & Co. and Cantor & Co.; 1835:253-384

2. Blackie GS. *Cretins and Cretinism,* A Prize Thesis of University of Edinburgh. Edinburgh: Maclachlan & Stewart and London: Simpkin, Marshall & Co.; 1855:31-35.

3. Inglis J. *Treatise on English Bronchocele: With a Few Remarks on the Use of Iodine and Its Compounds.* London: Longman, Orme, Brown, Green, and Longmans; 1838:23.

4. Scott H. Distribution of simple goitre in Derbyshire (Commentary). *The Indian Medical Gazette.* 1935:March,153.

5. Kelly FC, Snedden WW. Prevalence and geographical distribution of endemic goitre. In: *Endemic Goitre.* Monograph Series No. 44. Geneva: World Health Organization; 1960.

Chapter 5

Why Does Limestone-Source Water Cause Thyroid Disease?

Limestone is a term used by geologists. Chalk and lime are the terms used by the common man. In chemistry, limestone is called by its chemical name—calcium carbonate. When one drinks limestone-source water or hard water, one is taking excess calcium carbonate.

Calcium Carbonate disturbs acid–base balance in the body. Calcium carbonate makes the blood more alkaline than normal. The more alkaline blood results in all the symptoms that we see in hypothyroidism.

Before we discuss how excess calcium carbonate causes hypothyroidism symptoms, we will briefly discuss a few basic concepts of acids, bases, pH value, water in human body, and electrolytes.

i. Acids, Bases, and pH

Acid comes from the Latin word *acidus*, meaning *sour*. Acid is a substance that tastes sour. Everyday examples of acids are lemon juice, orange juice, tomatoes, and vinegar. Citric acid is the acid in lemons. Citric, malic, and ascorbic acids are the acids in oranges. Acetic acid is the acid in vinegar. Gastric acid in stomach is an example of an acid in human body.

Bases are the opposite of acids. They reduce the acidic property of acids. Everyday examples of bases are baking soda, antacid tablets, hand soap, bleach, and drain cleaner. The blood in human body is slightly basic or alkaline. The terms basic and alkaline are often used interchangeably.

The above description of acids and bases is a common man's description. In chemistry, acids and bases are defined in terms of concentration of hydrogen ions.

Ion

Ion is an atom or a molecule (a molecule is a group of atoms), with a net electrical charge.[1] A positive ion has more protons (positively charged particles) than electrons (negatively charged particles). A negative ion has more electrons than protons.

Hydrogen ion is a positive ion. It is represented by the chemical symbol H^+. When water dissociates, it dissociates into hydrogen ions and hydroxyl ions. Hydroxyl ion is a negative ion; it is represented by the chemical symbol OH^-.

When we put square brackets around the chemical symbol of an ion, it represents concentration of that ion in a solution: $[H^+]$ means concentration of hydrogen ions in a solution (e.g., blood), and $[OH^-]$ means concentration of hydroxyl ions in a solution (e.g., blood).

Definitions—Acid and Base[17(p11)]

The formal definitions of acids and bases in terms of hydrogen ion concentration, $[H^+]$, are:

> A solution is said to be acidic, or an acid, if its hydrogen ion concentration is greater than its hydroxyl ion concentration.
>
> A solution is said to be basic, or alkaline, if its hydrogen ion concentration is less than its hydroxyl ion concentration.

Therefore, hydrogen ion concentration, $[H^+]$, defines whether a solution is acidic or basic.

pH

The term pH stands for "power of hydrogen." pH measures the concentration of hydrogen ions (acid ions) in a solution. The more the hydrogen ions in a solution, the more acidic is the solution. The fewer the hydrogen ions, the more basic or alkaline is the solution.

pH is usually measured on a scale of 0–14. Substances with a pH value of 0 to 7 are acidic. Substances with a pH value of 7 to 14 are basic (alkaline). Substances with a pH value of 7 are neutral. The lower the pH value, the more acidic is the substance; the higher the pH value, the more alkaline is the substance. Table 5.1 lists a few examples of acids and bases and their pH values.

Table 5.1 Common substances and their pH values

Substance	**pH**
Hydrochloric acid	0.1
Gastric/stomach acid	2
Lemon juice	2.2
Cola	2.5
Vinegar	2.9
Orange/apple juice	3.5
Beer	4.5
Coffee/human urine	5
Tea/healthy skin	5.5
Milk	6.5
Pure water/distilled water	7
Healthy human saliva	6.5–7.4
Blood	7.35–7.45
Sea water	8
Hand soap	9–10
Bleach	12.5
Caustic soda	13.9

The pH scale is a *reverse* logarithmic (log) 10 scale. On a normal scale, a change from 7 to 8 would mean a change in one number. But on a logarithmic 10 scale, it represents a ten-fold change. In this case, since it is a reverse scale, it represents a reverse ten-fold change in hydrogen ion concentration. For example, a shift in pH from 7 to 8 represents a 10-fold *decrease* in hydrogen ion concentration, and a shift in pH from 7 to 9 represents a 100-fold (10×10) *decrease* in hydrogen ion concentration.

Limestone-source water that has a pH value of 8 would be 10 times more alkaline than pure water, which has a pH of 7. Limestone-source water that has a pH value of 9 would be 100 times more alkaline than pure water. In a survey in Goriganga river, in Pithoragarh district,[2] at the foothills of the Himalayas in India, the average pH value of water was 8.4; that is, the water in the river was 50 times more alkaline than distilled water. In another survey, in Ramganga river, in Pithoragarh district,[3] the pH value of water was 8.3; that is, thc water was 40 times more alkaline than pure water. Pithoragarh is the same region (discussed in the previous chapter) where John McClelland did his goiter and cretinism research.

Stomach acid, which has a pH value of 2, would be 100,000 times more acidic than pure water, which has a pH of 7. There is a five (5)-number difference between stomach acid and pure water. Therefore, on the reverse logarithmic 10 scale, it a difference of 10×10×10×10×10, i.e., 100,000 times.

Alkalinity

Alkalinity is not to be confused with alkaline. Alkaline means basic, i.e., opposite of acidic, whereas alkalinity is a measure of hardness. The more limestone in the water, the higher the alkalinity of the water.[4]

Table 5.2 Dissolved calcium carbonate, rather than starting pH of a solution, makes it difficult to make changes to pH

Water alkalinity (ppm of calcium carbonate)	Starting water pH	Sulfuric acid (ml) required to reduce water pH to 5
310	8.3	6
71	9.3	1.2

Credit: Buechel Tory.[4]

Table 5.2 shows that high alkalinity (measured in terms of dissolved calcium carbonate) makes it difficult to reduce the pH of water. Regardless of the starting pH, the higher the alkalinity (i.e., higher levels of dissolved calcium carbonate from limestone), the more acid is required to reduce the pH of water to 5. It is the level of alkalinity that determines how much acid is required to reduce the pH, not the starting pH. In Table 5.2 water with a higher pH does not require as much as acid as the one with a lower pH but with higher calcium carbonate.

Therefore, in the context of our discussion of thyroid disease, what is important is hardness of water, not the starting pH of water.

ii. Water in the human body

Till now, we have talked about water in the streams and mountains. Let us now talk about water *inside* the human body.

When we think of the human body, we usually do not think there is much water in it. We feel the human body is made of bones, muscles, skin, blood, and organs like heart, brain, liver etc., However, there is a large quantity of water in the human body. There are 42 litres of water in the body of a 70-kg (154-pounds) man. This is a very large quantity in comparison with the 2 litres of water that we usually drink every day. About 60% of body weight is water.

Water forms a significant portion of all organs. Brain is 75% water. Normally, when we think about the brain, we think about the fat matter in the brain, we do not think about the water/fluid in and around the brain. But notice how interesting this is: The brain is three-fourths water and one-fourth fat matter. The water in the brain is primarily in the cerebrospinal fluid surrounding the fat matter of the brain. This fluid itself is generated by the brain. This fluid is continuously replenished every six hours. Now, imagine the impact of drinking limestone-source water on the water in and around the brain.

Similarly, there is high water content in other organs. Lungs are 80% water, kidneys are 80% water, muscles are 80% water, heart is 70% water, skin is 60% water, and bones are 30% water. We may note that even bones, which are perhaps the strongest part of our body, are 30% water.

This water in the human body is not in pure water-form; it is in the form of fluids, mixed with electrolytes and nutrients. The kind of water we drink would ultimately reflect in the water in these organs and thus in the health or disease of these organs.

Water distribution inside the human body

The water in the human body is in two main places: inside the cells (*intracellular*) and outside the cells (*extracellular*).

Intracellular fluid is the fluid inside the cells. There are 28 litres of fluid inside various cells in the body. This fluid is located in all types of cells: nerve cells, muscle cells, skin cells, bone cells, and so on.

Extracellular fluid is the fluid outside the cells. There are 14 litres of fluid outside the cells. Of this, 11 litres are located in-between the cells called *intestinal space*. The remaining 3 litres are located in the blood plasma.

Figures 5.1 and 5.2 illustrate the location of water in the human body.

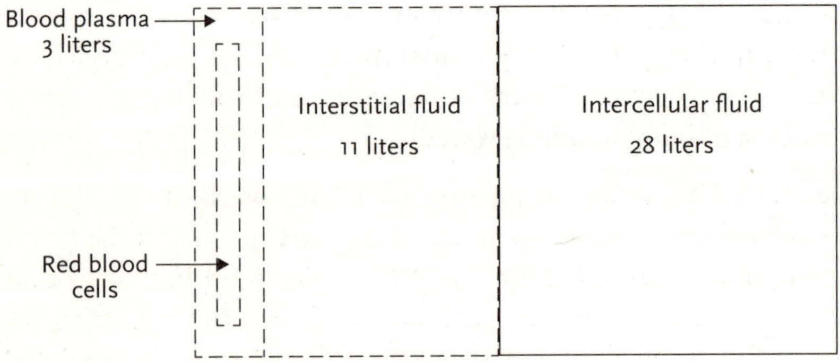

Figure 5.1 Fluid compartments and quantity of fluid in various compartments.

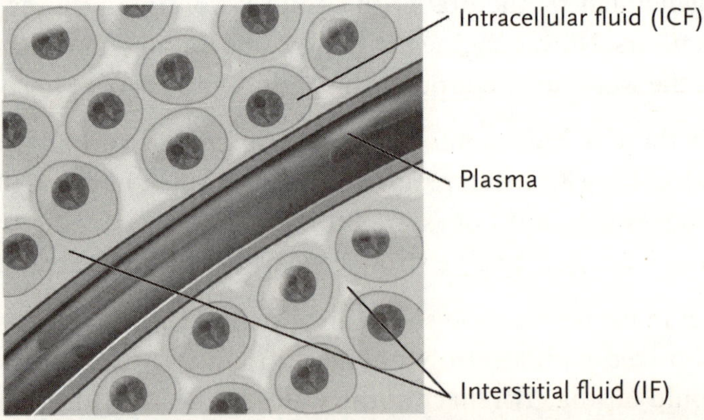

Figure 5.2 Image showing intracellular fluid, plasma, and interstitial fluid.

Blood plasma is a light-yellow-colored liquid in arteries and veins. Blood plasma is often called as plasma. Plasma does not include blood cells (red blood cells, white blood cells, and platelets).

About 55% of blood is plasma. The remaining 45% of blood is red blood cells, white blood cells, and platelets, which are suspended in the plasma.[5]

Plasma is 92% water, 7% proteins, and 1% electrolytes, hormones, carbon dioxide, oxygen, glucose, and blood clotting factors.[6,7]

Plasma plays an important role in maintaining blood pressure and volume, the proteins required for blood clotting and immunity, and the transport of electrolytes (sodium, chloride, potassium, calcium, bicarbonate, etc.) and hormones (thyroid hormones, insulin, adrenal hormones).

Plasma also plays a role in maintaining the correct pH balance in the body. It also transports the waste products generated in the cells of the body.

iii. pH Balance in the Human Body

Plasma is slightly alkaline, with a pH of 7.4. The plasma pH is maintained between 7.35 and 7.45. When plasma pH is less than 7.35, common in many critical illnesses, it requires admission to an intensive care unit.[8] When the pH is less than 6.8 or greater than 7.8, it often results in death.[9]

We may note that the normal plasma pH range is very narrow, just 0.10, from 7.35 to 7.45. Even in this normal range, plasma at the upper end of the normal range (pH 7.45) would be twice as alkaline as plasma at the lower end of the normal range (pH 7.35).

Extracellular fluid pH is maintained between 7.32 and 7.42. Intracellular fluid pH is maintained between 7 and 7.4. That is, extracellular fluid is more alkaline than intracellular fluid.

In arteries,[15] blood pH is maintained between 7.36 and 7.44. In veins, blood pH is maintained between 7.33 and 7.41. Such precision is required to meet the respective physiological functions, as arteries carry oxygenated blood and veins carry deoxygenated blood.

Similarly, the pH value varies in different tissues, depending on their function. For example, skeletal muscle[10,11] has a pH of 6.8–7.1. Within a cell, the pH value of different organelles[12,13] (an organelle is a subunit within a cell) can vary from 4.5 to 8. The pH within any organelle is tailored for its specific function. For example, lysosomes[12] have a relatively low pH of 4.5. Phagocytes also have a relatively low internal pH.[14] Since both these are degradative organelles that engulf and break down other substances, they require high internal acidity (i.e., low pH value) to perform their functions successfully.

In summary, pH balance is critical for both normal cell metabolism and function.[15] Even a minor deviation from the normal range can severely affect many organs and their functioning.

iv. Electrolytes

Sodium, potassium, chloride, magnesium, calcium, bicarbonate, and phosphate are examples of electrolytes. These electrolytes are mixed in the 42 litres of water in our body.

Electrolytes are important in the context of the thyroid gland. The following observation indicates their importance in the structure and function of the thyroid gland.

The weight of the thyroid gland in adults is 36–50 grams in inland areas, whereas it is between 20–30 grams near seacoast areas.[16] That is, the thyroid gland is roughly half the weight in people living near the seacoast than in those in inland areas. Near the seacoast, there is excess salt in the air. People living near the seacoast inhale salt into their lungs with every breath. Therefore, they take relatively more salt (through air) than people living inland. The chemical name of salt is sodium chloride. Thus, people living near the seacoast take in an excess of these two electrolytes, sodium and chloride. Over a long period, the excess of these two electrolytes changes the very structure of the thyroid gland, so much so that the weight of the thyroid gland is reduced to half. The reduction in the size of the thyroid gland would naturally affect its function. The body will have to adjust the other electrolytes to compensate for the excess of these two electrolytes.

Electrolytes, as their names says, have "electrical charge" in them. The word electrolyte is derived from the ancient Greek word *ēlectro,* meaning *related to electricity*, and *lytos* meaning *to be loosened.*

The chemical symbols and the electrical charges of various electrolytes are sodium (Na^+), chloride (Cl^-), bicarbonate (HCO_3^-), potassium (K^+), phosphate (HPO_4^{2-}), calcium (Ca^{2+}), and magnesium (Mg^{2+}). The positive symbol means the electrolyte has positive charge and the negative symbol means the electrolyte has negative charge.

The positively charged ions are sodium (Na^+), potassium (K^+), calcium (Ca^{2+}), and magnesium (Mg^{2+}). The negatively charged ions are chloride (Cl^-), bicarbonate (HCO_3^-), and phosphate (HPO_4^{2-}).

In blood plasma, the positively charged ions and negatively charged ions are in balance. Electrical neutrality is always maintained.

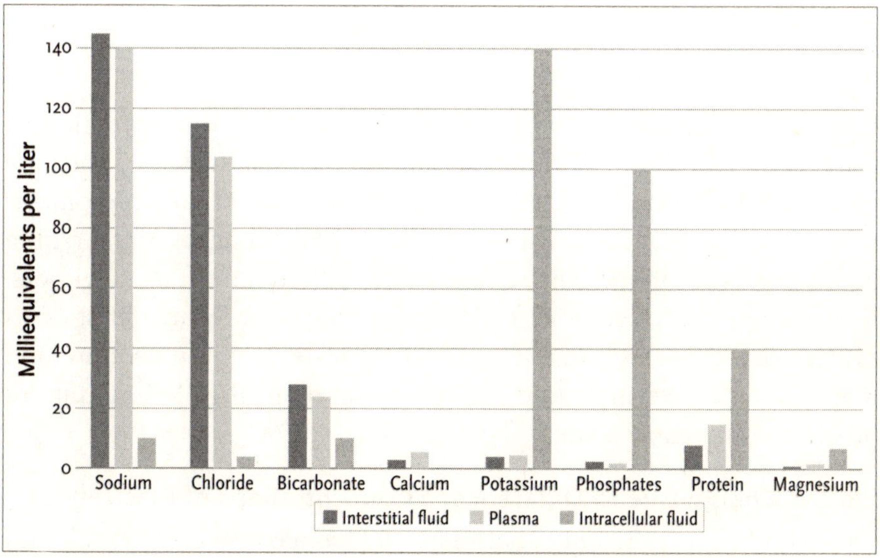

Figure 5.3 The concentrations of electrolytes in interstitial fluid, plasma, and intracellular fluid.

Figure 5.3 shows the dominant electrolytes in extracellular fluid (the four electrolytes to the left in the Figure) and the dominant electrolytes in intracellular fluid (the four electrolytes to the right in the Figure).

Extracellular fluid (interstitial fluid and blood plasma) is high in sodium and chloride, and low in potassium, magnesium, and phosphates. Intracellular fluid is high in potassium and phosphates, and low in sodium and chloride.

Bicarbonate is high in extracellular fluid and proteins are high in intracellular fluid.

Calcium is so low in intracellular fluid that it is not even registered as a bar in the graph. Calcium is 10,000 times less in intracellular fluid than in extracellular fluid.

Intracellular fluid contains high concentration of organic acids; extracellular fluid almost never contains organic acids.[17(p5)] Intracellular fluid, although lumped together, exists as tiny fluids in each of the trillions of cells. As different cell types are chemically different, their internal fluid will not be identical. But they share board common characteristics—high in potassium, phosphates, and magnesium, and low in sodium and chloride.

Like intracellular fluid, the interstitial fluid occurs as innumerable tiny pockets of solution in the interstices of all body tissues.[17(p6)] They are mostly in the form of very thin layers, of the order of one micrometer (1 μm i.e., one-millionth of a meter) or less. Each pocket of interstitial fluid (also called tissue fluid) is somewhat different from its neighbors. But overall, the interstitial fluid shares the same characteristics as discussed above—high in sodium and chloride, low in potassium and magnesium. Interstitial fluid has very low or negligible amounts of proteins and organic acids.

Electric Charge Due to Difference in Concentrations of Electrolytes

The significant difference between the concentrations of sodium and potassium inside and outside the cell cause the cell membranes (membrane is the outer boundary of a cell) to be electrically charged, with the positive charge on the outside the cell and the negative charge on the inside. This is illustrated in Figures 5.4 and 5.5.[18]

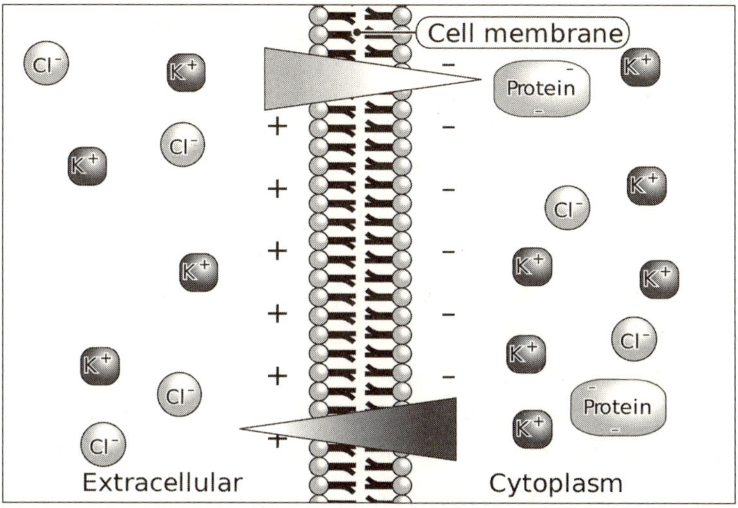

Figure 5.4 Differences in ion concentration on the opposite sides of a cell membrane produce a voltage difference[18]
Credit: Gibbs-Donnan-en.svg

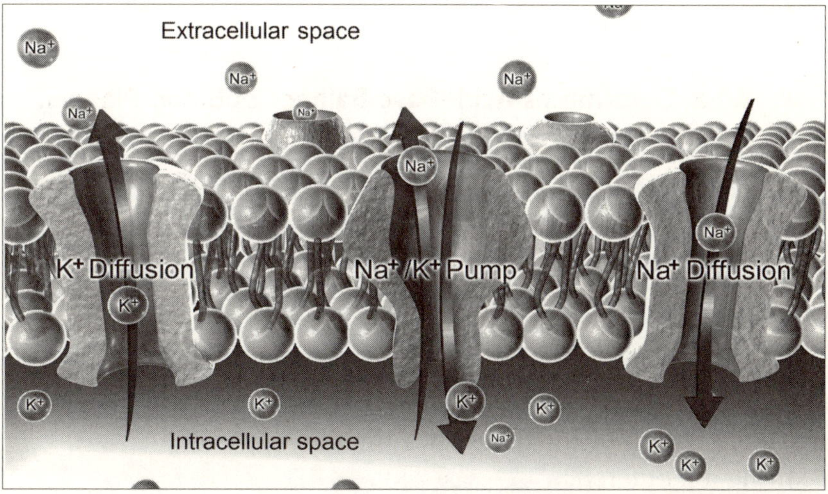

Figure 5.5 Sodium and potassium pumps in the cell membrane pump sodium and potassium in and out of cells[19]
Credit: Blausen.com, 2014

When there is an imbalance in the electrical charge, electrolytes are pumped in and out of the cell to bring the electrical charge into balance.[19]

v. Strong Electrolytes, Weak Electrolytes

When common salt (sodium chloride), is added to water, it completely dissociates into sodium ions and chloride ions.[17(p13)] There are no sodium chloride molecules left in the water.

Strong electrolytes are defined as those electrolytes that completely dissociate in a solution.[17(p14)] That is, the parent substance disappears completely when dissolved in water. In the above example, sodium ions and chloride ions are strong ions. The other common strong ions in biological solutions are potassium ions, magnesium ions, calcium ions, and a few organic acids such as lactate. Lactate ion functions as a strong acid because of the large dissociation constant of lactic acid.

Weak electrolytes are defined as substances that dissociate only partially when dissolved in water.[17(p14)] The molecules of the parent substance as well as the products of dissociation exist together in water. In body fluids, weak electrolytes are usually weak acids. Carbonic acid is an example of a weak acid.

vi. What Determines Acid–Base Balance of Blood Plasma?

Peter Stewart, a Canadian-born physiologist and Professor of Medicine at Brown University in the United States, made significant contributions to acid–base chemistry. We will draw on his insights on acid–base chemistry to understand how limestone-source water affects acid–base balance in plasma.

"Acid–base" means what happens to hydrogen ions in aqueous solutions. Per Peter Stewart, the hydrogen ion concentration or pH of any solution is dependent on three independent variables:

1. Strong ion difference
2. Partial pressure of carbon dioxide (Pco_2)
3. Total concentration of nonvolatile weak acids

Each of these variables independently affects the concentration of hydrogen ions in plasma, i.e., each of them affects the pH of plasma.

Strong Ion Difference

The hydrogen ion concentration of plasma (or plasma pH) depends to a large extent on the concentration of the strong ion difference in plasma.[17(p30)] Strong ion difference is the difference between the sum of strong positively charged base ions and the sum of the strong negatively charged acid ions.

The concentration of strong ion difference of plasma may be calculated as follows. The concentration of strong ion difference is denoted as [SID].

$$[SID] = \text{sodium } [Na^+] + \text{calcium } [Ca^{2+}] + \text{potassium } [K^+] + \text{magnesium } [Mg^{2+}] - \text{chloride } [Cl^-] - \text{lactate } [Lactate^-]$$

The square brackets in the above refer to the concentration of the respective ions in plasma. These concentrations are given in Figure 5.3. Therefore, we have:

$$[SID] = 140 + 5 + 4 + 1 - 107 - 2$$
$$[SID] = 41 \text{ milliequivalents per liter (mEq/L)}$$

This shows that when all electrolytes are at their normal concentration levels in plasma, the strong ion difference is 41 milliequivalents per liter (mEq/L).

As we can see from this definition, strong ion difference is the difference between positively charged ions and negatively charged ions. It is also the difference between base ions and acid ions. Therefore, it represents an excess of base over acid ions. In biological solutions, the strong ion difference is almost always positive.[17(p33)] In plasma, there is always excess of base ions over acid ions. This is why plasma is always alkaline, with a pH value of 7.4.

When the concentration of any electrolyte changes, the strong ion difference changes. And when strong ion difference changes, hydrogen ion concentration changes, i.e., pH changes. As the strong ion difference increases from the normal value of 41 milliequivalents per liter (mEq/L), the plasma pH increases, i.e., plasma becomes more alkaline. As the strong ion difference decreases from the normal value of 41, the plasma pH decreases, i.e., plasma becomes more acidic. Here we assume that the other independent variables (Pco_2 and the concentration of weak acids) remain the same.

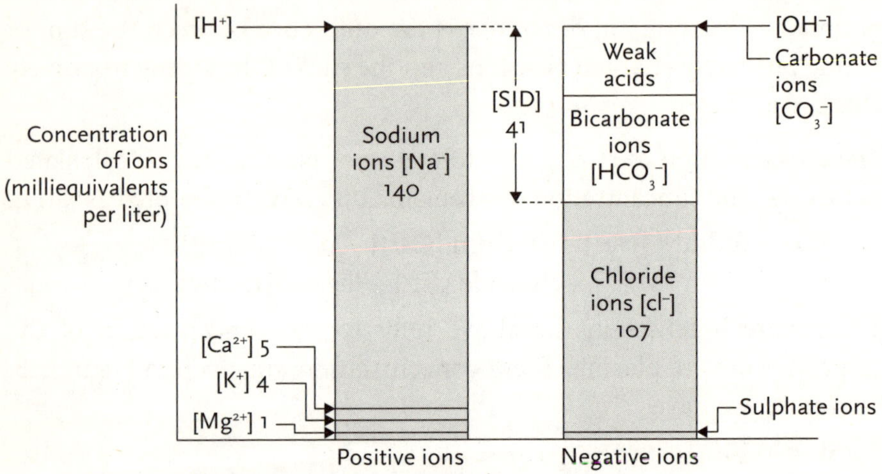

Figure 5.6 Concentration of ions in plasma

Figure 5.6 shows the concentration of ions in plasma. Here, $[H^+]$, $[OH^-]$, and $[CO_3^-]$ are so low that their concentration is represented by the thickness of the line.

In Figure 5.6, we note that

Strong ion difference [SID] = Bicarbonate $[HCO_3^-]$ + Proteins [weak acids]

Figure 5.7 on the next page indicates strong ion difference in intracellular fluid. This is for representation purpose only. The actual strong ion difference of intracellular fluid cannot be described quantitatively with the same degree of confidence in standard numerical terms as in the case of plasma or interstitial fluid.[17(p137)] Despite intracellular fluid being the largest fluid type in the body, it lies within cells and varies widely depending on the cell type. The strong ion difference in cells is very large compared to that of plasma or interstitial fluid, somewhere between 100 and 150 milliequivalents per liter (mEq/L).[17(p137)]

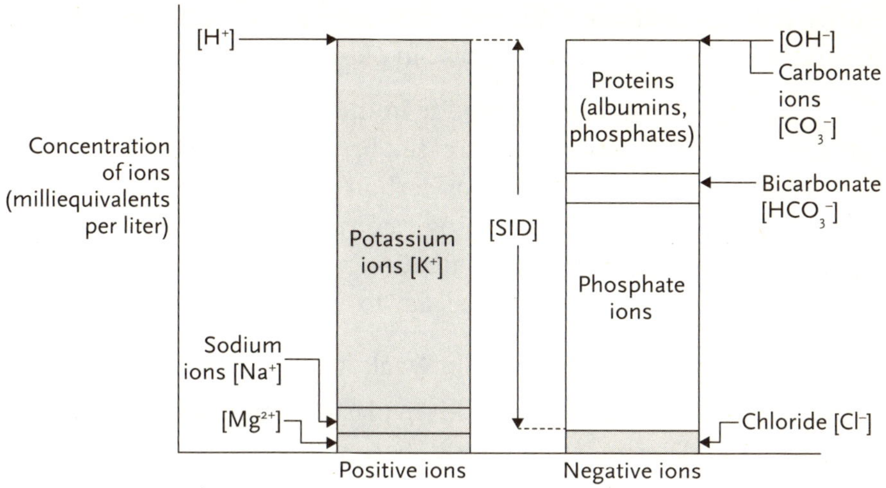

Figure 5.7 Concentration of ions in cells (or the intracellular fluid)

Partial Pressure of Carbon Dioxide (P_{CO_2})

Partial pressure of carbon dioxide (P_{CO_2}) is the second independent variable that affects acid–base balance in plasma. There is a direct relationship between partial pressure of carbon dioxide and hydrogen ion concentration. As P_{CO_2} increases, hydrogen ions (acid ions) increase and as P_{CO_2} decreases, hydrogen ions (acid ions) decrease.

Partial pressure of carbon dioxide (P_{CO_2}) in blood plasma indicates effectiveness of lung ventilation.[20] It is an indicator of respiratory function. It reflects carbon dioxide gas exchange in the lungs. It also reflects the amount of acid in the blood. It is measured in mm Hg units. In humans, the normal range is from 35 to 45 mm Hg. A value of more than 45 mm Hg indicates hypoventilation or reduced breathing rate. Value less than 35 mm Hg indicates hyperventilation or faster breathing rate. Under normal conditions, the plasma P_{CO_2} value is close to 40 mm Hg.

As the partial pressure of carbon dioxide in the plasma increases, it causes hypoventilation or a reduced breathing rate. During hypoventilation, the rate of removal of carbon dioxide from the blood is reduced. The reduced breathing rate increases the acidity of blood (or, in other words, reduces its alkaline nature). Thus, an increase in partial pressure of carbon dioxide leads to a decrease in plasma pH.

As partial pressure of carbon dioxide in the blood plasma decreases, it causes hyperventilation or an increased breathing rate. During hyperventilation, the rate of removal of carbon dioxide from the blood is increased.[21] The increased breathing rate reduces the acidity of blood (or, in other words, increases its alkaline nature). Thus, a decrease in partial pressure of carbon dioxide leads to an increase in plasma pH.

Total Concentration of Nonvolatile Weak Acids

The total concentration of weak acids in plasma is the third independent variable in the determination of acid–base status.

In acid–base chemistry, weak acids are often referred to as buffers. Buffers lessen the shock of drastic changes in acid–base behavior. Weak acids in fluid compartments are mainly proteins, and their concentrations normally vary by small amounts, and very slowly.[17(p76–77)] Examples of weak acids in plasma are albumin and phosphates.

vii. Principle of Electrical Neutrality

The sum of all positively charged ion concentrations equals the sum of all negatively charged ion concentrations in any macroscopic aqueous solution.[17(p16)] This is the principle of electrical neutrality (Figure 5.8).

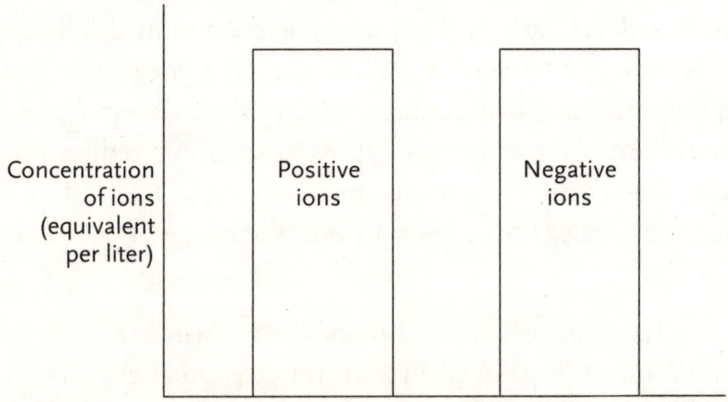

Figure 5.8 Concentration of positive ions equals the concentration of negative ions in a solution to maintain electrical neutrality.

Plasma, interstitial fluid, and intracellular fluid abide by this chemical principle. In these fluids, the total positive charge equals the total negative charge.

Whenever there are disturbances in electrical charge, electrolytes move from one fluid compartment to another, or the composition of electrolytes and buffers (such as bicarbonate and proteins) change to ensure that electrical neutrality is maintained at all times. For example, if one positive ion enters a cell, one positive ion must move out of the cell to maintain electrical neutrality. Or one negative ion must enter the cell along with a positive ion to maintain electrical neutrality.

The physical basis of this principle of electrical neutrality is Coulomb's law, which specifies that the very large electrical forces come into play whenever charge imbalance occurs.[17(p16)] For example, in a small sphere (1 millimeter radius) of solution, an excess of 0.0000001 Eq/L of positive ions (over negative ions) results in 400,000 V of electrical potential.[17(p16–17)] The chemically insignificant concentration difference of 0.0000001 Eq/L of excess positive ions produced an enormous electrical effect of almost half a million.[17(p17)]

Because ions in solution are free to move about, they will redistribute themselves very rapidly in response to such electrical forces, so that electrical neutrality is maintained, at all times to an extremely high level of precision.[17(p17)]

One reason strong ions are so important in understanding acid–base balance is that they are not involved in chemical reactions, so that their electrical charges are always present and have to be considered.[17(p167)] This is what strong ion difference [SID] does.

Hydrogen Ions Have Very Large Electrical Field Gradients in Their Neighborhood[17(p9–10)]

Hydrogen ion concentration in body fluids is extremely low, on the order of one ten-millionth to one hundred-millionth of an equivalent per liter.

Why are we so interested in the behavior of such rare species? As protons, hydrogen ions are very small, and therefore have a very high charge density. This in turn results in very large electric field gradients in their neighborhoods. They may, therefore, have important effects on other molecules in the solution around them, even at very low concentrations.

In particular, hydrogen bonds are important in the determination of macromolecular (proteins, carbohydrates, lipids, nucleic acids) structure and configuration, and their strengths would be particularly sensitive to local hydrogen ion concentrations. Partly for these reasons, enzyme (protein) activities are often significantly dependent on local hydrogen ion concentration.

Changes in hydrogen ion concentration have important effects on biochemical reaction rates simply because hydrogen ions are involved in so many biochemical reactions.

The hydrogen ion concentration, $[H^+]$, of blood in the veins is usually about 4.5×10^{-8} Eq/L (pH 7.35), while blood in the arteries is about 4×10^{-8} Eq/L (pH 7.4).

Table 5.3 Shows hydrogen ion and hydroxyl ion concentration at different pH values.

H^+ Concentration (mole/liter)	OH^- concentration (mole/liter)	pH
1	0.00000000000001	0
0.1	0.0000000000001	1
0.01	0.000000000001	2
0.001	0.00000000001	3
0.0001	0.0000000001	4
0.00001	0.000000001	5
0.000001	0.00000001	6
0.0000001	0.0000001	7
0.00000001	0.000001	8
0.000000001	0.00001	9
0.0000000001	0.0001	10
0.00000000001	0.001	11
0.000000000001	0.01	12
0.0000000000001	0.1	13
0.00000000000001	1	14

Hydrogen ion concentration above 1.2×10^{-7} Eq/L (pH 6.9) or below 1.6×10^{-8} Eq/L (pH 7.8) indicates life-threatening situations. Between these limits, wide variations can occur, sometimes very rapidly. This is what happens in hypothyroidism disease wherein hydrogen ion concentration is consistently low.

In this chapter and the subsequent chapters, we will discuss various topics in terms of changes in pH. However, we have to remember that whenever we talk about changes in pH, we are actually talking about changes in hydrogen ion concentration, and thus very large electrical field changes in their neighborhood. Therefore, when we say limestone-source water causes a change in plasma pH, we are saying that limestone-source water causes a change in hydrogen ion concentration in plasma, and hence, causes very large electrical changes in plasma.

viii. Why Does Limestone-Source Water Cause Hypothyroidism? Limestone-Source Water Increases Plasma pH

The impact of drinking limestone-source water is similar to the impact of taking an antacid tablet. Limestone-source water and antacid tablets are made of calcium carbonate. Antacids are popularly known as TUMS tablets in the United States. Antacid tablets are usually taken for excessive stomach acid. Antacids work by dousing the stomach acid. Similarly, calcium carbonate in limestone-source water douses the stomach acid. Every time one drinks limestone-source water, one is dousing the stomach acid. When stomach acid is thus continuously reduced, gastric cells in the stomach lining have to work continuously to produce more stomach acid, as the acid is required for normal digestion.

Chloride ions are required to produce stomach acid. Chloride ions are extracted from blood plasma and used by the gastric cells lining the stomach in the process of making stomach acid. This process of taking away of chloride ions from the plasma increases the strong ion difference in the plasma. Strong ion difference in plasma may be simply understood as the difference between the concentration of sodium ions and chloride ions, as the concentration of other electrolytes in plasma is quite low in comparison with these two electrolytes. An increase in strong ion difference causes a reduction in hydrogen ions. A reduction in hydrogen ions (acid ions) results in an increase in pH. Thus, calcium carbonate douses the stomach acid but ultimately results in an increase in plasma pH, i.e., makes plasma more alkaline than normal.

When one drinks limestone-source water, calcium carbonate ($CaCO_3$) dissociates into calcium (Ca^{2+}) and carbon dioxide (CO_2). Calcium from limestone-source water is absorbed through the intestine and enters the blood plasma. The excess calcium, a strong ion, further increases the strong ion difference in plasma. The increase in strong ion difference leads to a further increase in pH.

Carbon dioxide generated during dissociation of calcium carbonate increases the carbon dioxide levels in the plasma. The carbon dioxide (gas) turns into carbonic acid, and carbonic acid turns into bicarbonate. Thus, increase in carbon dioxide ultimately leads to an increase in bicarbonate, a base, which increases the plasma pH further.

Therefore, through multiple ways, limestone-source water increases the plasma pH, i.e., makes plasma more alkaline. However, we have seen previously, that plasma pH needs to be at 7.4 (or tightly regulated between 7.35 and 7.45) to perform many normal biological functions. On a cellular level, many essential cellular processes, metabolic enzymes, and cell transmembrane processes are highly pH sensitive.[22] When plasma pH goes beyond of this normal range, it results in metabolic alkalosis. Metabolic alkalosis is high concentration of bicarbonate (base ions) and low concentration of hydrogen ions (acid ions) in the blood plasma.[23] Many of the symptoms that we see in hypothyroidism are due to this metabolic alkalosis.

When the acid–base balance is disturbed by drinking limestone-source water, the body does not remain a bystander. It puts in place defense mechanisms to maintain the acid–base balance. The defense mechanism for metabolic alkalosis is through bicarbonate, lungs, and kidneys.

Bicarbonate

Drinking limestone-source water creates excess bicarbonate in the plasma. Usually, the higher the strong ion difference, the higher is the bicarbonate in plasma.

Bicarbonate is the most important buffer in defending acid–base balance in plasma. In addition to Stewart's approach, there is a traditional approach to acid–base chemistry. The traditional approach to acid–base chemistry is bicarbonate-centered. Per this approach, plasma pH is dependent on the plasma concentration of bicarbonate and the partial pressure of carbon dioxide. This approach underscores the importance of bicarbonate in regulating acid–base balance. The bicarbonate buffer system is responsible for 80% of the extracellular buffering.

Bicarbonate soaks up excess hydrogen ions (acid ions) to regulate acid–base balance. In any buffer system, the acid–base equilibrium is balanced by the presence of a weak acid and its related/conjugate base so that any excess acid or base introduced into the system is neutralized.[24] Carbonic acid is a weak acid, and bicarbonate is the related/conjugate base in our case. Carbonic acid changes into bicarbonate and vice versa to ensure that the plasma acid–base balance remains in the normal range. The following equation shows the buffering process in the bicarbonate buffer system.

$$\text{carbon dioxide} + \text{water} \rightleftharpoons \text{carbonic acid} \rightleftharpoons \text{bicarbonate} + \text{hydrogen ions}$$
$$CO_2 + H_2O \rightleftharpoons H_2CO_3 \rightleftharpoons HCO_3^- + H^+$$

The symbol $\rightleftharpoons$ means that the equation works both ways, from left to right and from right to left.

There is a huge amount of acid produced in the body during normal metabolism. Lactic acid is an example of acid generated during normal metabolism (e.g., physical activity or exercise produces a large amount of lactic acid). Bicarbonate neutralizes the acid produced during normal metabolism. Similarly, bases are produced during normal metabolism. Urea is an example of a base produced during normal metabolism, e.g., catabolism (breakdown) of proteins.[24] Bases are neutralized by carbonic acid. Thus, acids and bases produced during normal metabolism of the body are regulated by bicarbonate and carbonic acid respectively.

But when one drinks limestone-source water, one introduces an external factor that creates excess bicarbonate. Excess bicarbonate in plasma is produced by the increase in strong ion difference (attributable to less chloride in plasma). Thus, there is an overload of bicarbonate due to regular drinking of limestone-source water. The continuous overload of bicarbonate soaks up more acid ions than normal, resulting in perpetually more alkaline plasma than normal. The perpetually more alkaline plasma results in all the symptoms that we see in hypothyroidism.

Lungs

Lungs respond to an increase in plasma pH with a reduced breathing rate. The increase in plasma pH results in metabolic alkalosis; and the reduced breathing rate acts as a compensatory mechanism for metabolic alkalosis. The reduced beathing rate retains more carbon dioxide/carbonic acid in the plasma. This causes respiratory acidosis—a compensatory mechanism for metabolic alkalosis.

But the reduced breathing rate creates a problem. There is less oxygen available for normal metabolism, i.e., energy production inside the cells. Oxygen is required for energy production in the cell, in each of the estimated 37 trillion cells in the human body. But with reduced breathing rate, there is less oxygen and less energy production in the cells. The less energy production in cells results in a sluggish body and sluggish mind, the primary symptoms of hypothyroidism. Inadequately oxygenated cells also lead to increase in lactate, a strong acid, and thus a decrease in strong ion difference,[17(p154)] which may be another compensatory mechanism for metabolic alkalosis.

Carbon dioxide is generated in each cell of the human body during normal metabolism. About 360 litres of carbon dioxide is produced in the cells in a 24-hour period.[17(p87)] This carbon dioxide is transported to the lungs for exhalation. Carbon dioxide cannot be transported in gas form. Hence, carbon dioxide is converted into carbonic acid and the carbonic acid is then converted into bicarbonate. The bicarbonate is transported through blood to the lungs. In the lungs, bicarbonate is again converted into carbon dioxide and is eliminated through exhalation. Most of the carbon dioxide, about 70%, is eliminated through the bicarbonate form. With reduced breathing, more bicarbonate is retained in the blood plasma. Bicarbonate is a base. Thus, more base is retained in the blood, leading to increase in plasma pH. Thus, the compensatory mechanism of reduced breathing rate makes the blood even more alkaline. The acid–base balancing mechanism in the body goes into a vicious cycle. The body has to now deal with carbon dioxide generated during normal metabolism, carbon dioxide generated because of drinking limestone-source water, and carbon dioxide because of a reduced breathing rate (as a compensation for metabolic alkalosis). The body is overwhelmed. The plasma pH is now continuously higher than the normal pH. The higher plasma pH causes many symptoms that we see in hypothyroidism.

Kidneys

Kidneys play a primary role in metabolic-related acid–base imbalances—metabolic alkalosis and metabolic acidosis. Lungs, on the other hand, primarily play a role in respiratory-related alkalosis and acidosis.

Limestone-source water causes metabolic alkalosis. Kidneys address metabolic alkalosis by changing the rate of reabsorption of bicarbonate ions and strong ions.

A large quantity of blood, about 1000 mL, flows through kidneys per minute. From this huge quantity, the kidneys make about 1 mL of urine per minute. The rest of the blood is reabsorbed by the kidneys.

In their normal function, the kidneys reabsorb bicarbonate ions and strong ions from the blood when the blood passes through kidneys for filtration. The rate of reabsorption of strong ions affects the strong ion difference, which in turn affects plasma pH. Kidneys regulate plasma pH by differential reabsorption of sodium ions, chloride ions, potassium ions, and so on. Kidneys also regulate excretion of acid ions, specifically ammonia, to maintain plasma pH within the normal range.

When the plasma pH is high as in the case of drinking limestone-source water, the kidneys would either reduce the reabsorption of certain strong ions to bring down the strong ion difference or reduce reabsorption of bicarbonate to reduce the plasma pH. But kidneys are overwhelmed by the bicarbonate overload because of the regular drinking of limestone-source water. As a result, the kidneys are unable to bring the strong ions into balance or eliminate all the bicarbonate generated.

In addition, there may be other factors that affect the kidneys' role in maintaining plasma pH. These other factors are hormones of adrenal glands, such as angiotensin and mineralocorticoids. Adrenal glands are located just above the kidneys and are closely related to kidney function.

Angiotensin is a hormone that stimulates the release of another hormone, aldosterone, in the adrenal glands. Aldosterone promotes sodium retention by the kidneys. As more sodium is retained by kidneys, it leads to increase in strong ion difference (the increased sodium without a corresponding increase in chloride will increase the strong ion difference) and thus an increase in plasma pH.

Mineralocorticoids are the other hormones that are produced by adrenal glands. Mineralocorticoids influence the salt and water balance (electrolyte balance and fluid balance).[25] Thus, by playing a role in electrolyte balance, these hormones influence the acid–base balance. In hypothyroidism, constipation is a common symptom, the stools are hard, with little water/fluid in the stools. Therefore, these hormones, along with electrolytes, likely have a role in constipation. Kidneys too have a role in water/fluid balance, and hence likely have a role in constipation. Kidneys excrete excess acid in the process of achieving acid–base balance. Excess acid secretion by kidneys leads to diarrhea/loose stools, which is a characteristic symptom of hyperthyroidism. Since constipation is the opposite symptom of diarrhea, the kidneys may play a role in constipation by retaining more bicarbonate or less secretion of acids in hypothyroidism.

Another key symptom of hypothyroidism is fluid buildup in the face and body. Kidneys through their role in metabolic alkalosis, electrolytes through their role in acid–base balance and fluid balance, and hormones like mineralocorticoids through their role in electrolyte and fluid balance likely cause fluid buildup in the body, leading to thick and flabby skin, puffy face, and bloated body, as seen in hypothyroidism.

In summary, drinking limestone-source water makes the blood plasma more alkaline. The more alkaline blood plasma in turn causes the symptoms that we see in hypothyroidism. The human body has natural defense mechanisms to defend acid–base balance. The bicarbonate buffer system, lungs, and kidneys, through changes in their functioning, attempt to bring about acid–base balance. However, the defense mechanisms may not always be successful. Drinking limestone-source water every day creates an overload of bicarbonate and perpetually keeps the plasma pH high.

ix. High Plasma pH Changes Proteins' Shape and Structure

Water forms 60% of the human body. The next highest constituent of human body at 16% is proteins.

Normal protein functioning in the body requires that precise plasma pH be maintained. Many proteins have three dimensional structures. The extracellular proteins, such as the plasma proteins and membrane proteins, are very sensitive to pH.[26] Outside the acceptable range of pH, proteins become denatured (i.e., their three-dimensional structure is disrupted), causing enzymes to malfunction.

Let us assume the following diagram is the shape of an enzyme. An enzyme is a specific type of protein. A substrate is the substance on which an enzyme works on.[27] Enzymes can be thought of as factories that work on substrates to produce a chemical reaction. This process requires a normal plasma pH.

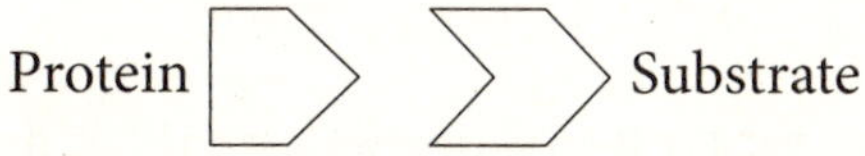

High plasma pH alters the shape of proteins. Drinking limestone-source water causes high plasma pH. Hence, the shape of the above protein may become changed as below.

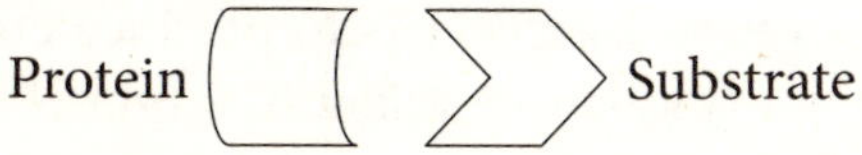

With the change in shape of the enzyme/protein, the enzyme/protein cannot work on the substrate. The chemical reaction cannot happen.

When the shape and structure of proteins are thus affected, their functioning is also affected. Since proteins form 16% of the body, proteins in all cells, tissues, and organs of the body are thus disrupted because of regular intake of limestone-source water.

Pepsin is an enzyme made in the stomach lining. Pepsin is required to digest proteins—meat, eggs, beans, pulses, lentils, seeds, dairy products, and so on.[28] In the absence of enough pepsin, protein digestion is impaired. This shows up as protein deficiencies in the body.

A high acidic environment is required to make pepsin. However, the stomach acid is reduced because of regular intake of limestone-source water. Hence, adequate pepsin may not be produced. In addition, the structure and shape of pepsin may become changed because of the high pH caused by drinking limestone-source water. Thus, digestion of all proteins in all foods may be affected. One may eat any amount of protein, but it may not be digested properly either because of inadequate pepsin enzyme or because of its disrupted shape and structure.

Skin, hair, and nails in the human body are made of proteins. Rough dry skin, brittle/weak hair, and broken nails, which are the characteristic symptoms of hypothyroidism, are due to the disruption in protein structure and impaired protein digestion.

Skin, hair, and nails are the visible forms of protein deficiency. There are a large number of other internal proteins whose shape may also be affected because of high plasma pH.

Hemoglobin

Hemoglobin is one such important internal protein. It carries oxygen in the red blood cells, from the lungs to every cell in the body. Although we normally say that blood carries oxygen from the lungs to rest of the body, it is actually this particular protein, hemoglobin, which carries the oxygen. The oxygen is then used by the cells to produce energy by the process of metabolism.[29] Metabolism is a key function of thyroid hormones. Thus, both hemoglobin and thyroid hormones work together in metabolism. Disturbance in either of them impairs metabolism.

Because of a high plasma pH, the shape and structure of the hemoglobin protein may also be affected. A healthy person has 12–20 grams of hemoglobin protein in 100 ml of blood. If the concertation is below this normal, he or she is said to have anemia. Anemia manifests as fatigue and is a key symptom of hypothyroidism. Therefore, the high blood pH affects the hemoglobin protein and its ability to carry oxygen, and this results in fatigue, the key symptom of hypothyroidism.

Hemoglobin also transports the carbon dioxide generated in cells. About 20%–25% of the carbon dioxide generated in the body is transported using hemoglobin. The high plasma pH, by affecting hemoglobin protein shape and structure, may also affect its ability to carry carbon dioxide. As more carbon dioxide is retained in the body, it disrupts the body metabolism and results in fatigue, a sluggish body, and a sluggish mind, the main symptoms of hypothyroidism.

Hemoglobin is also used as a buffer in maintaining acid–base balance. Since acid–base imbalance is caused by drinking limestone-source water, hemoglobin may be used up as a buffer to maintain the acid–base balance. This may lead to less availability of hemoglobin to discharge its normal function of carrying the oxygen and carbon dioxide in the blood.

Therefore, the hemoglobin protein may be affected in two ways—disruption of its shape and structure because of a high plasma pH and its reserves being used up as a buffer for countering acid–base imbalance.

We will now discuss three plasma proteins, which as their name says are present in the plasma (and not in the red blood cell). The function of these three plasma proteins is to transport hormones, lipids (fats and cholesterol), vitamins, and minerals, as part of their immune function.

Albumin

Like hemoglobin (150 grams/liter), albumin (70 grams/liter) is an important protein buffer that defends the body's acid–base balance.

Albumin is made in the liver. It accounts for 55% of all plasma proteins. It is a negatively charged protein/ion. When there is an increase in strong ion difference, it may result in an increase in weak acids such as albumin. But if an acid–base imbalance is caused by drinking limestone-source water, albumin may be used up as a buffer to maintain the acid–base balance, and so less albumin may be available to perform its normal functions.

The shape and structure of the albumin protein may also be affected because of the high plasma pH caused by drinking limestone-source water. Hence, albumin protein may not be optimally performing its primary function as a carrier of steroids, fatty acids, and thyroid hormones.

Globulin

Globulins make up 38% of plasma proteins. Globulin proteins are also made in the liver, with a few exceptions. They transport ions, hormones, and lipids as part of their role in immune system. High pH may affect the shape and structure of the globulin proteins and thus the discharge of their function as a carrier of hormones, which is of interest to us in the context of transport of thyroid hormones.

Fibrinogen

Fibrinogen accounts for 7% of plasma proteins. Fibrinogen is also made in the liver. It is essential for blood clotting, which is often delayed in hypothyroidism.

Histamine Intolerance

In hemoglobin and albumin protein buffering, histidine residues are involved. A histidine residue participates in forming a complex around a central atom or ion. For example, a histidine residue forms a complex around the central iron of a heme group.[30] Hemoglobin is quantitatively about six times more important in maintaining acid–base balance than the plasma proteins, as it is present in about twice the concentration and has about three times the number of histidine residues per molecule. (A hemoglobin molecule has 38 histidine residues.)

Since we are on the topic of histidine and proteins, a brief mention may be made about histamine in the context of thyroid disease.

Histidine is an essential amino acid that is used in the making of proteins. Histamine is derived from histidine. Histamine is a nitrogenous chemical substance that is involved in local immune responses. It regulates physiological functions in the gut, and acts as a neurotransmitter in the brain, spinal cord, and uterus.[31,32] Histamine is involved in the secretion of gastric juices, which (as we have noted earlier) is reduced by drinking limestone-source water, and is the starting point for hypothyroidism. Histamine is also involved in cell growth, cell differentiation, and wound healing. In the brain, histamine serves as an important neurotransmitter that regulates the circadian rhythm and promotes learning and memory.[33(p13)] Histamine intolerance is common in hypothyroidism. Low blood pressure, common in hypothyroidism, may be explained by the high histamine levels in the blood.

Almost every food contains histamine.[33(p5)] However, especially high histamine levels are found in aged/fermented food products like aged cheese, certain wines, frozen fish, spoiled fish, and sausages. Although histamine is important, the body has to also protect itself from too much of histamine. An enzyme called diamine oxidase, which is mainly made in the small intestine lining and found in the small intestine, liver, kidneys, and white blood cells, degrades the histamine.[33(p5)] When the body is unable to produce enough of this enzyme or if there is too much histamine, we have histamine intolerance. The hypothyroidism symptoms of lack of balance, vertigo, sea sickness (motion sickness) are symptoms of high histamine levels. As mentioned, histamine is involved in circadian rhythm, memory, and learning, which are known to be impaired in hypothyroidism. The high pH caused by limestone-source water changes the shape, structure, and function of enzymes and proteins, and in this case, the pH may affect the enzyme diamine oxide involved in degrading histamine. The process of acid–base buffering by hemoglobin and albumin proteins, which in turn involves histidine residues, may have role in high histamine levels in the body and the associated hypothyroidism symptoms.

In summary, limestone-source water causes an increase in plasma pH. This results in changes to the shape and structure of proteins, which in turn affects the entire body, as 16% of the body is made of proteins. The high pH disrupts functions of blood and plasma proteins and their role in acid-base buffering. The disruption in proteins such as hemoglobin results in fatigue, the main symptom of hypothyroidism, and a disruption of plasma proteins decreases their ability to carry hormones, steroids, and fatty acids, or to aid in blood clotting and other immune functions. The high pH and protein buffering may also lead to histamine intolerance and the associated hypothyroidism symptoms.

In this discussion, we have primarily focused on acid–base behavior in the context of one particular fluid compartment, i.e., plasma. However, as plasma circulates throughout the body, there is a continuous and rapid exchange of ions, electrolytes, and hormones among various fluid compartments (interstitial fluid and intracellular fluid). Acid–base homeostasis in plasma is rapidly equilibrated across fluid compartments.

x. Calcium Deficiency and Disruption

High pH causes calcium to bind to proteins, as calcium ions have a great propensity to bind to proteins.[34] As more calcium is bound to proteins, less free calcium may be available for other normal body functions. Calcium deficiency and disruption in calcium metabolism may explain the weak bones, rheumatic bone pains, muscle symptoms, and nervous symptoms in hypothyroidism.

Calcium also binds to bicarbonate,[38] a base, an excess of which is produced by drinking limestone-source water. This further reduces the free calcium available for normal body functions.

In North China, goiter researcher Bolt noticed a peculiar fact: the shells of hens' eggs in the vicinity of hard-water areas were much thinner than usual, and many of them were so deficient in lime salts as to leave the egg membranous in places.[35] Just like the hens, human beings and animals who drink limestone-source water show calcium deficiency symptoms. In cretinism, for example, the most visible symptoms are deformed bones. In goiter and hypothyroidism, rheumatic bone and joint pains and brittle bones are the key symptoms.

It may be appropriate to say that along with calcium deficiency, calcium metabolism is disrupted in hypothyroidism, as there is both weakness and deformity of bone. The deformity in bones may not be only due to deficiency but due to disruption in metabolism of calcium.

Calcium in Extracellular and Intracellular Fluid

Calcium is the most abundant mineral in the body.[36] When we think of calcium in the human body, we usually think of bones. Outside of bones and teeth, the majority of calcium is in the extracellular fluid. The total calcium in human body is 1,200 grams (42 ounces). About 99% of this calcium is in bones and teeth. Less than 1.5 grams (1,500 milligrams/mg) of calcium is in the extracellular and intracellular fluids. The calcium in the extracellular fluid is about 1050 mg. Of this, 700-mg is in the interstitial fluid and 350-mg calcium is in plasma.[37] The calcium in the intracellular fluid is 10,000 times less than the extracellular calcium. The concentration of calcium ions is the same as the concentration of hydrogen ions[17(p135)] in most cells in which it has been measured, on the order of 10^{-7}.

Importance of Calcium in Nerve and Muscle Functions

In addition to its role in bones, calcium plays an important role in the functioning of nerves and muscles. The muscle and nervous symptoms of hypothyroidism may be explained by the disruption in calcium metabolism.

Calcium is essential for muscle contraction. When a muscle is being used, calcium from outside the cell (extracellular fluid) is pumped into the cell (intracellular fluid) by the action of calcium pumps. When a muscle is at rest, calcium from inside the cell is pumped out into the extracellular fluid by the continuous action of calcium pumps.[38] Low calcium leads to various muscle related symptoms like spasms, cramps, and numbness. In severe cases, other muscle symptoms may result, shortness of breath, low blood pressure, and irregular heartbeat.[39]

Muscle related symptoms, spasms, cramps, and stiffness, seen in hypothyroidism are similar to the symptoms seen in calcium deficiency. Constipation seen in hypothyroidism may be due to inability of the colon muscles to contract and expand. Cross-eye/squint seen in cretinism in the endemic regions may also be due to inability of the eye muscles to contract and expand. Thus, the disruption in calcium metabolism leads to muscle symptoms seen both in calcium deficiency and hypothyroidism.

Similarly, in nerve cells, calcium enables transmission of a nerve impulse from one nerve cell to the next nerve cell. Calcium is pumped in and out of the nerve cell to enable the transmission of a nerve impulse. Thus, calcium is required in very minute quantities to enable nerve cells to do their job. When there is disruption of calcium metabolism, it leads to neurological symptoms.[39] The sluggish functioning of the brain, dulled senses, and deaf mutism in thyroid disease may be explained by impaired transmission of nerve impulses, in turn attributable to impaired calcium metabolism in the nerves and brain.

Calcium is also essential for release of neurotransmitters.[40] Neurotransmitters are brain chemicals. They play an important role in many brain functions such as decision-making, comprehension, memory, etc., Thus, limestone-source water and high blood pH disrupt calcium metabolism, which in turn cause disruption in the release of neurotransmitters and the associated brain functions.

Importance of Calcium in a Cell

Calcium exists in each of the estimated 37 trillion cells in the human body. Calcium is located both on the cell membrane and inside the cell. It maintains cell membrane stability and permeability. We have seen that when muscles contract, there is an increase in the calcium concentration inside the cell. When the muscle is at rest, the calcium is pumped out of the cell. A cell has channels and pumps in the cell membrane that regulates the flow of calcium between the intracellular fluid and the extracellular fluid. Most intracellular calcium is in a complex and sequestered form in the cell membrane.[38] The free intracellular calcium level depends on energy-requiring processes, which remove calcium from the cell or sequester it in cell organelles.[38] In short, the functioning of every cell is dependent on calcium as it is involved as a gatekeeper in the cell membrane. If calcium is allowed to accumulate in a cell because of the failure of a calcium pump, this accumulation leads to cell death. The accumulation of calcium in a cell is one of the effects of low oxygen.

The sodium channels in the cell membranes of nerve cells and muscle cells have an even greater sensitivity to changes in the calcium concentration of the extracellular fluid.[41] Relatively small decreases in the plasma calcium levels cause these sodium channels to leak sodium into the nerve cells, making them hyperexcitable, thus causing spontaneous muscle spasms.[41,42]

Importance of Calcium in Proteins

As noted earlier, calcium ions have a great propensity to bind to proteins.[43] When calcium attaches to a protein, it changes the distribution of electrical charges on the protein, with the result that the three-dimensional structure of the protein is altered.[43,44] Thus, limestone-source water causes disruption of proteins by increasing plasma pH and by attaching calcium to proteins.

Protein structures so disrupted show symptoms in skin, hair, nails, hemoglobin, and plasma proteins. According to Ayurveda, the ancient Indian medical science, hair and nails are the byproduct (*mala*) of bones (*asthi*).[45] This shows calcium metabolism was long recognized in the health of hair and nails.

Bone Deformities in Cretinism

If we look at the bone deformities in cretinism, some observations may be made. There is a lack of symmetry in overall bone development. The head is disproportionate in size to the rest of the body. The summit of the head is flat. The end of long bones is enlarged; for example, the knee and elbow joints, which are located at the end of long bones, are enlarged. The knees are bent inward as in rickets disease. The feet are flat. All these symptoms show that calcium is deposited more in certain places and less in certain places. This may not mean calcium deficiency. It may mean that normal calcium metabolism and function is disrupted. Why is this happening?

There is bone marrow (red bone marrow) below the enlarged knee and elbow joints. Red bone marrow is the place where stem cells make new red blood cells, white blood cells, and platelets. The enlarged joint may reflect a problem in the red bone marrow. We know that red blood cells are reduced and malformed in hypothyroidism, resulting in fatigue. There is also a disproportion in the type of white blood cells. In hypothyroidism, there is a reduction in number of one type of white blood cells called lymphocytes, usually from 30% to 18% of total white blood cells.[46] There is an increase in the number of another type of white blood cells called eosinophils, usually from 2%–3% to 11%–16% of white blood cells.[46] Platelets are also made in the red bone marrow. Platelets help in blood clotting. In hypothyroidism, there is usually delayed blood clotting. This shows the link between red bone marrow, red and white blood cells, and hypothyroidism symptoms. Therefore, the deformed bones in cretinism may be due to impairment in red bone marrow, although impaired calcium metabolism may also play a role.

In summary, limestone-source water makes the blood more alkaline, which disrupts calcium metabolism and new blood cell generation in bone marrow, leading to bone-related symptoms in hypothyroidism. The disrupted calcium metabolism also causes the muscle, nerve, and neurological symptoms of hypothyroidism. While the disruption of normal metabolism (energy-producing process) in cells explains each of these symptoms, the disruption of calcium metabolism is the additional factor that explains these symptoms.

xi. Temperature and pH

There is an inverse relationship between temperature and pH. As the temperature drops, the pH increases. As the temperature rises, the pH falls.

In the human body too, the blood pH varies inversely with body temperature.[47]

The average blood pH is 7.4 at the normal body temperature of 37 °C.

When blood pH is 7.35, i.e., when the blood is more acidic, the body temperature is high at 40 °C.

When blood pH is 7.45, i.e., when the blood is more alkaline, the body temperature is low at 34 °C.

The relationship between temperature and pH may explain the constant symptoms of chill and cold-feeling in hypothyroidism.

xii. Electrolytes and Thyroid Disease

In the previous section on electrolytes, we gained a basic understanding of electrolytes. In this section, we will briefly look at electrolytes and their functions in the context of thyroid disease symptoms.

The fact that salt weather near the seacoast reduced the size of the thyroid gland by half shows how important a role electrolytes play in the structure and function of the thyroid gland.

Electrolyte Imbalance Symptoms and Thyroid Disease Symptoms Are Similar

Electrolytes are not restricted to any one part of the body. They are spread throughout the 42 litres of fluid in the body, from the brain to intestines, to bones and various organs. Therefore, the symptoms of electrolyte imbalance are spread throughout the body, just as in thyroid disease, the symptoms are spread throughout the body, from the brain to an individual cell.

Electrolyte balance is maintained by intake of electrolyte-containing foods and is regulated by various hormones. Imbalances can develop by consumption of too little or too much of electrolytes. The kidneys play an important role in regulating the electrolyte levels in the body by reabsorbing electrolytes and flushing out excess electrolytes. In the context of our subject, electrolyte imbalance is produced because of drinking an excess of limestone-source water and the resulting disruption in the balance of other electrolytes.

The most common symptoms of electrolyte imbalance and their relation to thyroid disease symptoms are described now.

Acid–Base Balance

As discussed earlier, electrolytes control and regulate acid–base balance through their role in strong ion difference. The electrolytes sodium and chloride are the main determinants of strong ion difference in plasma and interstitial fluid. The electrolytes potassium and phosphate are the main determinants of strong ion difference in intracellular fluid.

Other electrolytes such as calcium and magnesium also influence strong ion difference and thus the acid–base balance. Acid–base imbalance is the immediate cause of thyroid disease symptoms. This shows the importance of electrolytes in thyroid disease.

Muscles

Muscles are activated by electrolyte movements between the interstitial and intracellular fluids. For example, the contraction and expansion of muscles is dependent on calcium levels inside and outside the muscle cells. Even potassium and sodium are involved in muscle function.

Electrolyte imbalance leads to weak muscles, muscle cramps, and numbness of muscles, which are also the symptoms in thyroid disease.

Nerves

Both muscles and nerves are electrical tissues. Imbalance in electrolytes leads to imbalance in electrical activity in the muscle and nerve tissues.

Bones

Calcium, which is involved in bone metabolism, is an electrolyte. Magnesium and phosphate are the two electrolytes that are involved in the metabolism of calcium, through their action on vitamin D absorption. Thus, indirectly, these two electrolytes are also involved in bone function.

Imbalances in any of these electrolytes may cause weak and deformed bones, which are a common symptom in hypothyroidism.

Fluid Balance

Sodium and potassium are the two main electrolytes involved in fluid balance. Hypothyroidism symptoms like puffy face, bloated body, and constipation are due to impaired fluid balance and electrolyte balance.

In summary, it may be said that electrolytes, through their roles in acid–base balance, muscles, nerves, nervous system, bones, and fluid balance, have a key role in hypothyroidism symptoms.

Summary

We have discussed many topics in this chapter. The summary is limestone-source water makes the blood more alkaline, which in turn causes many symptoms of hypothyroidism.

We may also note that the body tries to achieve a balance at many levels. The body tries to achieve electrical neutrality by balancing positive charged ions and negative charged ions in the fluid compartments. In order to achieve the electrical neutrality and acid–base balance, electrolytes are moved in and out of fluid compartments. In order to achieve acid–base balance, the body temperature is adjusted. The secretion of various hormones is increased or decreased in response to changes in electrical neutrality, acid–base balance, electrolyte balance, and body temperature. The functions of various organs such as the lungs and kidneys are modified to bring about the acid–base balance. Thus, the body continuously tries to balance electrical neutrality, acid–base level, body temperature, electrolytes, hormones, and the functions of various organs. In this process of balancing various systems, an external input like limestone-source water causes acid–base imbalance, ultimately leading to hypothyroidism symptoms.

References

1. Ion, Wikipedia. https://en.wikipedia.org/wiki/Ion. Accessed June 8, 2022.

2. Kumar A. DIEL Variations of physico-chemical factors at BARAM in glacial fed mountainous Goriganga river of Uttarakhand, India. *Res J Chem Sci.* October 2014:4(10):20-23.

3. Seth R, Mohan M, Singh P, et al. Water quality evaluation of Himalayan rivers of Kumaon region, Uttarakhand, India. *Appl Water Sci.* 2016:6:137-147.

4. Buechel T. Water alkalinity vs. pH—What's the difference? Pthorticulture. https://www.pthorticulture.com/en/training-center/water-alkalinity-vs-ph/. Published Nov 9, 2021. Accessed May 8, 2022.

5. Body fluids and fluid compartments. Opentextbc. https://opentextbc.ca/anatomyandphysiologyopenstax/chapter/body-fluids-and-fluid-compartments/. Accessed May 31, 2022.

6. The importance of plasma in blood. red cross blood. https://www.redcrossblood.org/donate-blood/dlp/plasma-information.html. Accessed May 8, 2022.

7. Blood plasma. Wikipedia. https://en.wikipedia.org/wiki/Blood_plasma. Accessed May 8, 2022.

8. Allyn J, Vandroux D, Jabot J, et al. Prognosis of patients presenting extreme acidosis (pH <7) on admission to intensive care. *J Crit Care.* 2016;31:243-248. In: Higgins C. *Extreme Acidosis and Mortality—A Retrospective Clinical Study*. Acute Care testing. https://acutecaretesting.org/en/journal-scans/extreme-acidosis-and-mortality---a-retrospective-clinical-study. Accessed on May 8, 2022.

9. Blood pH. Harper College. http://dept.harpercollege.edu/chemistry/chm/100/dgodambe/thedisk/bloodbuf/zback.htm. Accessed on May 8, 2022.

10. Brandis K. Regulation of intracellular hydrogen ion concentration. Acid–base physiology. Anaesthesia Education Website. In: Intracellular pH. Wikipedia. https://en.wikipedia.org/wiki/Intracellular_pH. Accessed on May 8, 2022.

11. Madshus IH. Regulation of intracellular pH in eukaryotic cells. *Biochem J.* February 1988:250 (1):1-8. In: Intracellular pH. Wikipedia. https://en.wikipedia.org/wiki/Intracellular_pH. Accessed May 8, 2022.

12. Asokan A, Cho MJ. Exploitation of intracellular pH gradients in the cellular delivery of macromolecules. *J Pharm Sci.* April 2002;91 (4):903–13. In: Intracellular pH. Wikipedia. https://en.wikipedia.org/wiki/Intracellular_pH. Accessed May 8, 2022.

13. Proksch E. pH in nature, humans, and skin. *J Dermatol.* September 2018:45 (9):1044-1052. In: Intracellular pH. Wikipedia. https://en.wikipedia.org/wiki/Intracellular_pH. Accessed May 8, 2022.

14. Nunes P, Guido D, Demaurex N. Measuring phagosome pH by ratiometric fluorescence microscopy. *J Visualized Exp.* December 2015:(106):e53402. In: Intracellular pH. Wikipedia. https://en.wikipedia.org/wiki/Intracellular_pH. Accessed May 8, 2022.

15. Hamm LL, Nakhoul N, Hering-Smith KS. Acid-Base Homeostasis. *Clin J Am Soc Nephrol.* 2015;10(12):2232-2242. doi:10.2215/CJN.07400715

16. McCarrison R. *The Thyroid Gland in Health and Disease.* New York: William Wood. 1917:4.

17. Stewart P. *How to Understand Acid–Base. A Quantitative Acid–Base Primer for Biology and Medicine.* New York: Elsevier; 1981.

18. Gibbs-donnan-en.svg: Biezl (derivative work: Looie496). Commons.wikimedia.org. https://commons.wikimedia.org/w/index.php?curid=8969169. Accessed May 8, 2022.

19. Sodium-potassium pump and the diffusion between extracellular fluid and intracellular fluid. Wikipedia. https://en.wikipedia.org/wiki/Extracellular_fluid#/media/File:Sodium-potassium_pump_and_diffusion.png. Accessed May 8, 2022.

20. pCO_2 Wikipedia. https://en.wikipedia.org/wiki/PCO2. Accessed May 8, 2022.

21. Hyperventilation. Britannica. https://www.britannica.com/science/hyperventilation. Accessed May 8, 2022.

22. Hamm LL, Nakhoul N, Hering-Smith KS. Acid-base homeostasis. *Clin J Am Soc Nephrol.* 2015;10(12):2232-2242. doi:10.2215/CJN.07400715.

23. Goldfarb DS, Kenny J-ES (2019). Chapter 79 – Metabolic alkalosis. In: Lerma EV et al. (eds.) *Nephrology Secrets* (4th ed.). Elsevier; 2018.

24. Bicarbonate buffer system. Wikipedia. https://en.wikipedia.org/wiki/Bicarbonate_buffer_system. Accessed May 8, 2022.

25. Mineralocorticoid. Wikipedia. https://en.wikipedia.org/wiki/Mineralocorticoid. Accessed June 3, 2022.

26. Macefield G., Burke D. Paraesthesiae and tetany induced by voluntary hyperventilation: Increased excitability of cutaneous and motor axons. *Brain*. 1991:114 (1): 527-540. doi:10.1093/brain/114.1.527 In: Acid Base Homeostasis. Wikipedia. https://en.wikipedia.org/wiki/Acid-base_homeostasis. Accessed May 8, 2022.

27. BiologyVittles. Bicarbonate Buffer System. YouTube. https://www.youtube.com/watch?v=N3oh0ApQRiE&list=PLlRAAoNKYzT-F5mZxjxEGd6QFojoIit1cl&index=5&t=301s. Accessed May 8, 2022.

28. Pepsin. Britannica. https://www.britannica.com/science/pepsin. Accessed May 8, 2022.

29. Hemoglobin. Wikipedia. https://en.wikipedia.org/wiki/Hemoglobin. Accessed May 8, 2022.

30. Histidine residue. ScienceDirect. https://www.sciencedirect.com/topics/chemistry/histidine-residue. Accessed May 8, 2022.

31. Marieb E. *Human Anatomy and Physiology*. San Francisco: Benjamin Cumming; 2001:414. In: Histamine. Wikipedia. https://en.wikipedia.org/wiki/Histamine. Accessed June 3, 2022.

32. Nieto-Alamilla G, Márquez-Gómez R, García-Gálvez AM, Morales-Figueroa GE, Arias-Montaño JA. The histamine H3

receptor: structure, pharmacology, and function. *Mol Pharmacol.* 2016:90 (5): 649-673. In: Histamine. Wikipedia. https://en.wikipedia.org/wiki/Histamine. Accessed June 3, 2022.

33. Jarisch R, Wantke F, Raithel M, Hemmer W. Histamine and biogenic amines. In: *Histamine Intolerance. Histamine and Seasickness.* Jarisch R (ed.) Springer; 2012:5.

34. Stryer L. *Biochemistry* (4th ed.). New York: W.H. Freeman; 1995. pp. 255-256, 347-348, 697-698 in: Extracellular Fluid. Wikipedia. https://en.wikipedia.org/wiki/Extracellular_fluid. Accessed May 8, 2022.

35. Kelly FC, Snedden WW. Prevalence and geographical distribution of endemic goitre. *Endemic Goitre.* Monograph Series No. 44. World Health Organization; 1960:175.

36. Peacock M. Calcium metabolism in health and disease. *Clin J Am Soc Nephrol.* 2010:5(Suppl 1):S23–S30 In: Calcium Metabolism. Wikipedia. https://en.wikipedia.org/wiki/Calcium_metabolism. Accessed May 8, 2022.

37. Schaafsma G. Calcium in extracellular fluid: Homeostasis. In: Nordin BEC (eds) *Calcium in Human Biology.* ILSI Human Nutrition Reviews. London: Springer; 1988. https://doi.org/10.1007/978-1-4471-1437-6_10.

38. Edwards SL. Maintaining calcium balance: Physiology and implications. *Nursing Times*; 2005:101(19)58-61.

39. Walls RM, Hockberger RS, Gausche-Hill, M. *Rosen's Emergency Medicine: Concepts and Clinical Practice.* Philadelphia, PA: Elsevier; 2018:1516-1532.

40. Electrolyte Balance. Open Text BC. https://opentextbc.ca/anatomyandphysiologyopenstax/chapter/electrolyte-balance/. Accessed May 8, 2022.

41. Armstrong CM, Cota G. Calcium block of Na^+ channels and its effect on closing rate. *Proc Natl Acad Sci USA.* March 1999:96

(7):4154-4157. doi:10.1073/pnas.96.7.4154. In: Extracellular Fluid. Wikipedia. https://en.wikipedia.org/wiki/Extracellular_fluid. Accessed May 8, 2022.

42. Harrison TR. *Principles of Internal Medicine* (3rd ed.). New York: McGraw-Hill. pp. 170, 571-579. In: Extracellular Fluid. Wikipedia. https://en.wikipedia.org/wiki/Extracellular_fluid. Accessed May 8, 2022.
43. Stryer L. *Biochemistry (Fourth ed.)*. New York: W.H. Freeman and Company; 1995:255–256, 347–348, 697–698. In: Extracellular Fluid. Wikipedia. https://en.wikipedia.org/wiki/Extracellular_fluid. Accessed May 8, 2022.
44. Macefield G, Burke D. Paraesthesiae and tetany induced by voluntary hyperventilation. Increased excitability of human cutaneous and motor axons. *Brain.* 1991:114 (Pt 1B) (1): 527–40. doi:10.1093/brain/114.1.527.
45. Uniyal Parmita. Ayurveda expert on tips to boost calcium levels naturally. https://www.hindustantimes.com/lifestyle/health/ayurveda-expert-on-tips-to-boost-calcium-levels-naturally-101649756788621.html. Published April 12, 2022. Accessed April 14, 2022.
46. Kocher ET. Concerning pathological manifestations in low-grade thyroid diseases. Nobel Lecture, December 11, 1909. https://www.nobelprize.org/uploads/2018/06/kocher-lecture.pdf. Accessed: May 8, 2022.
47. Constable P. Why is blood pH regulated? *Critical Care Nephrology* (2nd ed.); 2009. In: Blood pH. ScienceDirect. https://www.sciencedirect.com/topics/medicine-and-dentistry/blood-ph. Accessed May 8, 2022.

Chapter 6

Soil Type and Thyroid Disease

Water gets its quality from the rocks and soil it flows through. In this chapter, we will see if *limestone soil* could also cause thyroid disease.

About 88 years ago, in 1934, H. Scott, a British doctor, and S. P. Gupta, an Indian doctor, made a few observations on the relationship between soil type and thyroid disease.[1] The observations were made at the foothills of the Himalayas, in the superendemic areas of Gonda and Gorakhpur districts of Uttar Pradesh, the largest state in India.

In the Padrauna locality in these districts, the soil was of two types—Bangar and Bhat. The distribution of goiter in this locality corresponded with the distribution of Bangar and Bhat soils. Bangar soil covered about 25% of the locality and yielded a produce of superior quality. Bhat soil was of two types—pure bhat soil and sandy bhat soil. The produce of pure bhat soil was of medium quality. The produce of sandy bhat soil was of the lowest quality. Bhat soil is limestone soil. For a moment, forget whether these soils cause disease in man. Bhat soil (limestone soil) is not good even for plant health, as it produced low quality crop. On the other hand, bangar soil is good for plant health, as it produced superior quality crop.

Superendemic goiter areas in the Padrauna locality were limited to limestone soil. Limestone soils of Uttar Pradesh have soft lime in subsoils to an extent of 30%–40%. Padrauna Chaoni was a village situated both on bangar soil and bhat soil. The portion of the village on bangar soil was practically free of goiter, while the portion on limestone soil showed many goiter cases. Many wells in bangar soil were reported to possess the property of curing goiter.

There were exceptions to the above general rule. There were villages on bangar soil with a goiter rate of about 30%–35%. On the other hand, there were villages on limestone soil with a goiter rate under 5%. Probably, these exception villages in limestone soil got their drinking water from a nonlimestone source. Similarly, the villages on bangar soil with 30%–35% goiter rate probably got their water from a limestone source. As we have seen from the research of McClelland, the source of drinking water is the primary cause of thyroid disease. Soil is likely secondary to water in causing thyroid disease. Food grown on limestone soil probably causes thyroid disease over a long period of time.

Limestone Soils Have Excess Calcium

In 1934, Scott et. al. observed that limestone soil in the Padrauna area had a calcium content of 32%. Bangar soil, on the other hand, had a calcium content of 2%.[2] In normal soil, the calcium content was 0.3%. That is, the calcium content of limestone soil was 100 times the calcium content of normal soil.

Elsewhere, in the marshy limestone tract of Gorakhpur in Bahraich, Gonda, and Basti, the soil had a calcium content of 9%, i.e., the calcium content of limestone soil was 30 times the calcium content of normal soil.

Limestone Soils Are Deficient in Many Minerals and Micronutrients

Excess lime (calcium carbonate) in soil makes the soil alkaline. The increase in alkaline nature of soil (increase in pH) affects the health of plants. This is similar to how increase in the pH of blood and body fluids by drinking limestone-source water causes symptoms of hypothyroidism in men and women. The increase in soil pH results in low nitrogen, phosphorous, zinc, and iron.[3] The increase in pH causes deficiency of all other minerals and micronutrients.

Farmers with acidic soils usually apply lime (calcium carbonate) to improve the productivity of their farms. However, excessive use of lime can decrease the availability of many essential plant minerals, such as boron, iron, zinc, copper, manganese, magnesium, phosphorous, and molybdenum.[4] Grass and food grown on such soils will be deficient in these minerals and micronutrients. When animals and human beings eat food grown on such soils, they are bound to be deficient in these minerals and micronutrients.

Foot and Mouth Disease Thrives in Limestone Soil

Foot and mouth disease is a disease that affects animals like cattle, sheep, goats and pigs. The disease causes a high fever lasting two to six days, followed by blisters inside the mouth and on the feet. The blisters may rupture and cause lameness; hence, the name foot and mouth disease. The disease can sometimes be fatal. The cause of the disease is generally considered to be an infection from a *virus*, a foot-and-mouth-disease virus. But note the observations below and the importance of limestone soil in the cause of this disease.

In 1939, Peters, a German veterinarian, presented to the Veterinary Association of Stuttgart a report on the geographical distribution of foot-and-mouth disease in Württemberg, Germany.[5(p140)] In sandy, granitic, and gneissic soils, less than 10% of the animals were affected by foot-and-mouth disease, whereas in limestone soils, 35%–40% of the animals were affected by foot-and-mouth disease. Sometimes even 70%–80% of animals were affected in certain districts.

Similar observations were made in France. The Assistant Director of Agriculture Services at the Loir-et-Cher region, France, observed that foot-and-mouth disease did not develop to any great extent on the sandy soils in the Sologne area, in the center of France, and in the Finistere region of France, where granitic soils were widespread.[5(p141)]

The above observations in Germany and France show that limestone soil and foot-and-mouth disease share a common geography. Therefore: Is the cause of foot-and-mouth disease a virus or limestone soil?

We know from the previous chapter that excess limestone causes an increase in pH. An increase in pH in the blood of animals feeding on grass grown on limestone soil creates a conducive environment for various infectious bacteria/viruses to thrive. Further, as mentioned earlier, limestone soil is deficient in many minerals and micronutrients. When animals feed on grass grown on such deficient soils, the animals likely become deficient in those nutrients. Hence, the immune system of the animals becomes weak, and the foot-and-mouth disease virus easily attacks such weak animals. Therefore, although the virus is the immediate cause of foot-and-mouth disease, limestone soil creates a conducive environment for the virus to attack the cattle.

Grains and food grown on limestone soil are likely to have a similar effect on human beings. Food grown on limestone soils similarly causes an increase in blood pH in man, and such food is also deficient in various minerals and micronutrients. Our immune system then gets weak and prone to various infectious attacks, just like the cattle feeding on grass grown on limestone soil.

Modern Agriculture

"Soil makes the man" is an old adage. Health of man depends on health of soil. In modern agriculture, "man makes the soil" through use of synthetic fertilizers. Modern agriculture disturbs the balance of soil by excessive use of select synthetic (man-made) fertilizers.

The synthetic fertilizers used by modern farmers usually contain three main minerals, nitrogen, phosphorous and potassium. These three minerals, together with calcium, sulfur, and magnesium are called macronutrients, as these are required by plants in relatively large quantities. There are other minerals known as trace minerals, which are needed for soil and plant health in low concentrations, in a few parts per million or even less. These are copper, zinc, iron, manganese, molybdenum, selenium, nickel, cobalt, boron, and so on. In modern farming, these other minerals and trace minerals do not get the same attention as the big three. For example, selenium is very important in thyroid health. Selenium concentration is higher in the thyroid gland than in any other organ in the body and, like iodine, selenium has important functions in making the thyroid hormone.[6] Usually, selenium does not get the attention that iodine gets in thyroid health. A soil deficient in selenium is likely to have an impact on thyroid health. Excessive focus on a few minerals in modern agriculture disrupts the fine balance of minerals in soil and grass. Such mineral imbalance leads to imbalance in amino acids (proteins) in the grass. And when animals consume grains from such grass, the mineral balance in blood of the animal is disturbed. Thus, imbalance in the soil creates imbalance in the blood.

As an example, we will now see the impact of excess of one mineral—potassium—on soil health and animal health.

Impact of Potash (Potassium) Fertilizer on Grass

Potash refers to potassium compounds commonly used as fertilizer in agriculture. In 1954, at the Potassium Symposium organized by the International Potash Institute, the following findings were reported.[7] When potash was applied to grass at the rate of 230 lb/acre, the quantity of grass produced increased 200%, from 6,900 to 21,000 lb/acre. The potassium content in the grass increased from 1% to 3%. However, the magnesium content in grass decreased from 0.55% to 0.41%. The decrease in magnesium may look small, but the decrease relative to the potassium content of grass is significant. In relative terms, the potassium content of the grass is now 600% more than magnesium content of grass before potash fertilizer application. The farmer may feel good about the increase in quantity of the grass produced. But the significant decrease in the magnesium content of the grass relative to its potassium content leads to imbalance in the blood of the animal eating such grass.

Impact of Excess Potash Fertilizer on Animal

Animals suffer from *grass tetany*, a disease which occurs in cattle when the magnesium content is low relative to the potassium content in the blood of the animal.

Grass tetany is a metabolic disorder primarily characterized by muscle symptoms. Cattle affected by acute grass tetany have stiffening of muscles and violent jerking convulsions (spasms/tremors/shaking). They show unusual alertness such as staring and keeping their heads and ears in an erect position. They have a staggered gait/walk and have twitching skin, especially on the face, ears, and flanks. They lie down and get up frequently. There is an increase in body temperature and respiratory rate.[8] However, clinical signs are not always evident before the animal dies.[9] The connection between tetany and thyroid disease is that some of these symptoms are quite similar to those of hyperthyroidism in human beings.

The immediate cause of grass tetany is deficiency of magnesium in the blood of the animal. Giving magnesium injections to affected cattle immediately gives relief.

But it is not absolute deficiency of magnesium which causes tetany. It is the deficiency of magnesium and calcium relative to potassium that causes tetany. Dutch scientists showed through statistics that when potassium content in the grass was less than two times the total of the magnesium and calcium content, tetany was unknown. But when potassium content in grass was three times or more than the total magnesium and calcium content in the grass, 17% of the cattle were affected by grass tetany. This shows the negative effects of putting excess potash fertilizer. The excess potash fertilizer causes an imbalance in the soil, resulting in imbalance in the blood of the animal (through the intermediary of the grass).[10(p413)]

There are a few other interesting observations regarding grass tetany. The grass tetany period is early spring, when the season is transitioning from winter to spring, and in few cases early autumn. In early spring, the number of cases increase five days after the temperature starts to rise from below 14 °C. During the warmer summer months, there are practically no tetany cases.

Another observation was that in tetany-causing grasses, extremely high nitrogen was noted, while sodium was found to be consistently low.[10(p424–425)] Tetany was more common in high nitrogen soils than in limestone soils. Soil that was slightly to moderately acidic showed more grass tetany cases.[10(p417)] Several European researchers noted that heavy applications of nitrogenous and potassic fertilizers, particularly when used together, caused lower serum magnesium levels and an increase in the incidence of grass tetany. When nitrogen and potassium are too high in the herbage, the commonly accepted safe magnesium content of 0.2% in herbage might prove inadequate.[10(p422)]

Another observation was that the greatest number of deaths in tetany occurred within a week or two after calving, but some occurred just before the calving date[10(p416)]. Grass tetany occurred when the energy demand (e.g., high milk production) exceeded energy intake. The high protein/low energy nature of pastures, particularly in spring and autumn, was noted as the possible cause of animal disorders. Especially, the high protein grass favored the development of grass tetany.[10(p412)] In tetany-causing grasses, the soluble carbohydrate, which was taken as a relative measure of energy-producing constituents of the herbage, was found to be low.[10(p428)] Thus, carbohydrate was low and protein/nitrogen was high in tetany-causing grasses.

From the above discussion, we can see that it is not simple magnesium deficiency that causes grass tetany; rather, it is excess of potassium relative to magnesium and calcium in the blood of the animal, excess nitrogen and low sodium in soil and herbage, acidic soils, high phosphorus relative to calcium and magnesium,[10(p432)] excess crude protein in herbage due to excess nitrogen, deficient carbohydrate/glucose, excess insulin, and excess protein in the blood of the animal. All these factors contribute to tetany. This shows that soil affects the grass, the grass affects the blood and results in disease in the animal.

Human beings also are affected by tetany. Tetany symptoms are muscle cramps, spasms, and tremors. The muscles contract involuntarily, i.e., without intention or involvement. Tetany is the result of overly stimulated muscles. Tetany is usually caused by low calcium. Hypoparathyroidism causes low calcium. Hypoparathyroidism is deficient secretion of the parathyroid hormone. An excess of phosphate (high phosphate-to-calcium ratio) can also trigger spasms. Low levels of magnesium can also lead to tetany in human beings. All these observations show how closely linked are the functioning of muscles and nerves (since muscles get their instructions from nerves) with various electrolytes—calcium, potassium, magnesium, phosphorus, and various hormones—parathyroid hormone, thyroid hormone (which is also involved in calcium metabolism). Thus, electrolytes and hormones are closely related in their functions. Imbalances in minerals in soil lead to imbalance in electrolytes and hormones, which lead to muscular symptoms like tetany. The above discussion further confirms the involvement of electrolyte imbalances in thyroid disease, as discussed in the previous chapter.

While the above example of tetany is a symptom of hyperthyroidism, it shows that soil can affect thyroid gland. Similarly, limestone soil affects thyroid health and results in hypothyroidism as shown by the research of Scott and others. However, the impact of soil on thyroid health could be over a long period unlike the immediate impact of limestone water.

In summary, the fact that limestone soil has 30 to 100 times more calcium carbonate than normal soil leaves no scope for doubt that soil does have an impact on health of plant/grass and hence on the animal/man consuming produce of limestone soil. The impact is through an imbalance in electrolytes in the blood of the animal/man.

References

1. Scott H, Gupta SP. The distribution of goitre in the united provinces. *Ind Jour Med Res.* 1934;XXI(3):652-653.

2. Scott H, Bhatia BB, Lal RS, Rai KC. The distribution and cause of endemic goitre in the united provinces. *Ind Jour Med Res.* 1931;18(4):1059-1085.

3. Food and Agriculture Organization of the United Nations. Management of calcareous soils. https://www.fao.org/soils-portal/soil-management/management-of-some-problem-soils/calcareous-soils/en/. Accessed May 8, 2022.

4. McCleod CC. Effects of limes on soil acidity. In: Trotter B. *Soil Minerals – The Key to Farming Wealth and Your Own Health*. Zealand; 2005.

5. Voisin A. *Soil, Grass and Cancer*. London: Crosby Lockwood & Son Ltd.; 1959.

6. Selenium Factsheet for Health Professionals. National Institute of Health. https://ods.od.nih.gov/factsheets/Selenium-HealthProfessional/. Updated March 26, 2021. Accessed May 8, 2022.

7. Walsh T. Potassium Symposium 1954. In: Voisin A. *Soil, Grass and Cancer*. London: Crosby Lockwood & Son Ltd.; 1959:47-49.

8. Allison C. Controlling Grass Tetany in Livestock. Nmsu.edu. https://aces.nmsu.edu/pubs/_b/B809/. Updated January 2003. Accessed May 8, 2022.

9. Grass tetany. Kansas State Univ. Research and Extension, Forage Facts series. In: Grass Tetany. https://en.wikipedia.org/wiki/Grass_tetany. Accessed May 8, 2022.

10. Metson AJ, Saunders WMH, Collie TW, Graham VW. Chemical composition of pastures in relation to grass tetany in beef breeding cows. *NZ J Agri Res*. 1966;9(2). DOI: 10.1080/00288233.1966.10420793.

Chapter 7

Food and Thyroid Disease

Food and thyroid gland influence each other. Food influences the functioning of the thyroid gland, and thyroid gland influences the metabolism of food.

i. Influence of Food on Thyroid Gland

Food Grown on Limestone Soil

We have discussed this topic in the previous chapter in the context of animals. In man, food grown on limestone soil probably has a bigger role in the cause of mild thyroid disease than do specific food items. Limestone soil is more alkaline and is deficient in many minerals and trace elements. Grains grown on such soil disturb the pH balance in the blood of man because of mineral/electrolyte imbalance in the grains. Over a long period, consuming grains grown on limestone soil makes man susceptible to thyroid disease. This likely happens over a very long period. Even when drinking limestone-source water, it takes a very long time for a person to develop goiter. McClelland noted that goiter takes over six years or longer to develop in a few individuals. In the case of food grown on limestone soil, it could take an even longer time for a person to develop into goiter. But mild thyroid disease symptoms could develop over a much shorter time. Vegetables, pulses, beans, and oil seeds grown on limestone soil likely have a detrimental effect on the thyroid gland.

Food Processing

The way grains are processed may have an impact on the thyroid gland. Traditionally, grains (rice, wheat) were processed using stone and wooden motor and pestles. With industrialization, grains began to be processed using machines. Machine processing of grains removes B vitamins, minerals, and fat in the outer layer (bran) of grains. The excessive heat generated during the machine milling process leads to significant loss of nutrients. Polishing and refining processes, which are common to modern milling of grains, further remove minerals from the grains.

Rice was never polished in traditional processing with wooden motor and pestle. Only the husk (the hard outer layer) was removed. With the arrival of new machine-milling processes in the late 1800s, rice was not only processed to remove the husk but was also polished. Polished rice is a problem in the context of thyroid disease. In his experiments, Robert McCarrison, a British thyroid researcher in India, fed pigeons an exclusive diet of polished rice.[1(p39)] Pigeons so fed died in large numbers from invasion into the blood by certain microorganisms of the *Escherichia coli* group, which normally inhabit birds' intestines, but which may normally (in health and healthy diet conditions) exist harmlessly.[1(p39)] There were significant changes in the thyroid gland of pigeons with feeding of polished rice. The thyroid gland was enlarged, there was loss of colloidal substance[1(p39)] (a substance which is required for producing thyroid hormones), and evidence of thyroid cell-exhaustion and pronounced wasting/decline in function. The thyroid gland changes in such cases were largely due to an infection. But the infection itself was due to the deficiency in food, which in this case was due to *polished* rice. Polished rice affects a number of organs in the body, thyroid gland is just one of the organs. Under the influence of polished-rice diet, the thymus gland reduces in size significantly, the reproductive organs undergo pronounced wasting/decline in function, and the liver undergoes great enlargement.[1(p39)]

Similarly, modern milling process of wheat (and white bread made from refined wheat flour) creates mineral imbalance in the blood of man and likely has an impact on the thyroid gland. The endosperm portion of the wheat grain (the center layer of grain) makes up about 80% of the wheat grain volume. The white flour made of endosperm is preferred in modern cooking because the products made from the endosperm have milder flavor and smoother texture. The balance of the wheat grain is composed of the bran and the germ which, tend to be coarser. With the invention of the roller-milling system in the late 1800s, the bran and the germ could be removed. In 70% extracted refined wheat flour there is, in comparison with whole-wheat-flour, a 70% loss of potassium, 87% loss of magnesium, 50% loss of calcium, 60% loss of iron, 65% loss of copper, and 70% loss of zinc.[2(p53)] The commonly consumed white bread is made from such refined wheat flour.

The absolute loss of minerals is not the only problem. Milling disturbs the relative proportion of various minerals. In 70% extracted wheat flour, the potassium content is reduced by 70%, whereas the magnesium content is reduced by 87%.[2(p53)] This results in a relative excess of potassium in comparison with magnesium in the wheat flour. The ratio of potassium to magnesium more than doubles, from 3.4 to 8.[2(p53)] Similarly, the ratio of potassium to total of calcium and magnesium increases by 30% (from 2.6 to 3.3).[2(p53)] As we have seen in the previous chapter, excess potassium relative to magnesium and calcium is harmful to the health of the cattle. Similarly, low magnesium content in the blood causes convulsions (tremors, spasms, shakings) in humans. These are hyperthyroidism symptoms. This shows that excessive processing of grains can have a negative impact on the health of the thyroid gland.

This is not a speculative hypothesis. In the years of poverty and shortages that followed World War II, a serious wave of goiter overwhelmed Germany and Austria. It developed not only in the classical, endemic goiter regions, but also in many areas where it had never been seen before. One of the causes attributed for this wave of goiter was the new method of wheat flour processing using machines, which had then been recently introduced in these countries. However, the form thyroid disease noted in these cases was hyperthyroidism.

Usually, when discussing thyroid disease, the focus is on certain foods that cause goiter (e.g., cabbage, cauliflower). However, these food items are consumed occasionally and in relatively less quantity; hence these foods are not likely to cause a permanent damage to the thyroid gland. On the other hand, excessive processing of staple grains could have a more lasting negative impact on the thyroid gland as staple grains are consumed with every meal.

Thus, overprocessing of grains leads to hyperthyroidism symptoms, rightly so because overprocessing of grains may make the grains more acidic, and excess acid is the cause of hyperthyroidism. As the subject of this book is hypothyroidism, we can draw an inference from the above discussion that the general health of the thyroid gland is affected by consuming overprocessed grains. Although overprocessed grains may not cause hypothyroidism, consuming such grains might worsen preexisting hypothyroidism and delay recovery.

Food Cooked in Limestone Source Water

An observation in my ancestral village in India is that food cooked in limestone source water/hard water takes a significantly longer time to cook. This is starkly observed when cooking lentils such as red gram, which takes unusually long to cook in hard water. Food absorbs water during the cooking process. In this case, limestone-source water is absorbed in the cooked food. Consuming food cooked in limestone-source water would ultimately make blood more alkaline and cause hypothyroidism symptoms.

Quantity of Food and Nutrition

In 1934, in the Gonda and Padrauna areas at the foothills of the Himalayas in India, the quantity and quality of food did not appear to have a role in causing goiter. Many poor people were not affected by goiter although they were taking the same diet as people who were affected by goiter.[3(p652)] On the other hand, a few well-to-do people who lived on good quality food were affected by goiter.[3(p652)] American missionaries and their children living in the same locality, who likely had access to better quantity and quality of food, were affected by goiter.[3(p652)] These observations show that the quantity and quality of food did not have a major role in the cause of goiter.

However, in the endemic regions at the foothills of the Himalayas in Uttar Pradesh, India, there was an increase in goiter rate after food famines, and new centers of goiter were observed. Researchers in widely separate parts of the world reported an increase in the incidence of endemic goiter after the World Wars I and II. Such an increase apparently occurred in Eastern Europe, Western Europe, England, Taiwan, and New Zealand.[4] These goiters were more similar to hyperthyroidism-type goiters than hypothyroidism goiters. Various explanations have been offered for these epidemics, including changes in the food, water supply, deficiency of vitamin A, and iodine. However, no direct evidence was brought forward in support of these various claims.

In 1908, Robert McCarrison, undertook a series of experiments on goats, with the object of transferring goiter from man to goats by means of water infected with fecal matter.[1(p36)] It was observed during the course of these experiments that animals that received a poor diet and were ill-nourished showed a higher percentage of thyroid changes than those that were well fed, all other factors remaining the same in both classes.[1(p36)] Similar observations were made in ill-nourished puppies, calves, and lambs in certain parts of America.[1(p36)]

Therefore, given these conflicting observations, we may conclude that malnutrition has a negative effect on the thyroid gland. Adequate nutrition offers some protection against disease. Limestone-source water may cause disease in thyroid gland irrespective of the nutrition status, as in the case of the well-to-do people and American missionaries at the foothills of the Himalayas.

Exclusive Meat Diet

Herbivores show a high iodine content in the thyroid gland compared to carnivores. In dogs, it was found that the iodine-containing colloid substance in the thyroid gland may be made to disappear by feeding them on an exclusive meat diet. Under an exclusive meat diet, the gland's reserve of iodine-containing colloid substance is soon exhausted, the vesicles become empty, smaller in size, and shrunken into various shapes, the intervascular tissue becomes relatively increased—all changes indicative of an attempt at increased activity on the part of the thyroid gland, which is followed by degenerative changes in the parenchyma cells, atrophy, and a diminution in size of the whole gland.[1(p37)] All these technical terms simply mean that the thyroid gland is adversely affected by an exclusive meat diet.

In rats fed an exclusive diet of meat, the gland continued in a state of active secretion, with loss of stored-up colloid; and if the diet was continued, pathological effects were produced.[1(p30–31)] Cell exhaustion from continued hyperactivity may lead to symptoms of thyroid disease. Hence, a mixed diet containing an abundance of vegetables may be the natural and most appropriate food for man.[1(p30–31)] The reason an exclusive meat diet is harmful to the thyroid gland may be due to the excessive protein and nitrogen content of the meat diet. We have seen evidence of this in the previous chapter, where an excess of protein and nitrogen leads to tetany and hyperthyroidism symptoms in cattle.

Goiter-Causing Foods

Every food that we eat has some problem or the other in it. Grains, vegetables, and fruits develop a small quantity of poison or antinutrients to protect themselves from grazing animals. For example, the hard cover/husk over grains protects the grains from being consumed by grazing animals. When grazing animals consume grains with husk, the husk creates a gastrointestinal discomfort in the grazing animal, thus dissuading the animal from further grazing the grains. Thus, plants create these toxins to protect themselves against predators.

The common foods known to cause goiter because of toxic substances in them are sweet potato, cassava, millets, soy, peanuts, and cruciferous vegetables like cabbage. There are certain substances in these foods, which when consumed without proper preparation or cooking may cause goiter. These substances are thiocyanate, cyanogenic glucosides, and flavonoids. We need not go into details of these technical terms.

But if these food items were so problematic, our ancestors would not have continued consuming them. Our ancestors were smart. They found ways to minimize the harmful effects of these substances. Over thousands of years, our ancestors have found ways to process and cook these foods to minimize the harmful effects of these toxins. Techniques like fermentation and boiling were used to make these foods edible and less goiter-causing. Most of these foods—cassava, millets, soy, and cabbage—were traditionally fermented before eating. In places where there is already the problem of limestone-source water, consumption of these food items could aggravate disease in the thyroid gland.

Sweet Potato

In Gonda, at the foothills of the Himalayas, the poor laborers consumed sweet potato and maize in winter and the millets jowar and bajra in summer.[3(p653)] Many local people in Gonda believed that goiter was caused by consuming sweet potato. But researchers Scott and Gupta observed that in the western part of Gonda and Padrauna, no sweet potato was produced or consumed, and that rice and maize formed the main diet. Yet, these places were affected by goiter. So, the researchers concluded that sweet potato did not cause goiter.

The local people in Gonda were right to an extent. We know today that sweet potato has a goiter-causing substance in it. In endemic areas where people were already susceptible to goiter (attributable to limestone-source water), a goiter-causing food like sweet potato could aggravate the assault on the thyroid gland. The above observations show that limestone-source water is the primary cause of goiter/hypothyroidism, and that food (sweet potato in this case) is likely a secondary cause.

Cassava

Not many people in the United States or other developed countries eat cassava. But worldwide, 800 million people depend on cassava as their primary staple food in Africa, South America, and Southeast Asia.[5] In tropical countries, it is the third-largest food source, after rice and maize. Cassava, yams, and sweet potatoes are the important sources of food in the tropics, because these crops can grow in poor soils and in areas with low rainfall.

Cassava has cyanide. Cyanide is the poison that we see in the movies; spies and terrorists consume cyanide to avoid torture when they get caught by their enemies. In technical terms, cassava contains two *cyanogenic glucosides, linamarin* and *lotaustralin*. Cyanogenic glycosides are natural plant toxins that are present in several plants, most of which are consumed by humans.[6] Cyanide is formed following the hydrolysis of cyanogenic glycosides, which occurs during crushing of the edible plant material, either during consumption or during processing of the food crop. The cyanogenic glucosides are decomposed by *linamarase*, a naturally occurring enzyme in cassava, which detoxifies the cyanogenic glycosides.[7] The cyanide level of cassava varies from about 75 to 350 ppm (parts per million), but can be up to 1000 ppm or more, depending on the variety, plant age, soil condition, fertilizer application, weather, and other factors.[8]

Long-term low-level exposure to cyanide from improper preparation of cassava is associated with the development of goiters and ataxia, a nerve-damaging disorder that renders a person unsteady and uncoordinated.[9,10] The reliance on cassava as a food source and the resulting exposure to the goitrogenic effects of thiocyanate was responsible for the endemic goiters seen in Southwestern Nigeria.[11,12] Societies consuming cassava as staple food have devised ways to address these toxic effects of cyanogenic glycosides. In West Africa, cassava was traditionally fermented. The cassava roots are peeled, put into water for three days to ferment, then dried, and cooked. The fermentation process reduces the level of antinutrients, making cassava a more nutritious food.[13]

The inference we can draw from this is that consumption of cassava leads to general disruption of the many bodily functions, and thyroid gland is one of them.

Millets

Millets are small cereal grains. Just like cassava, millets are a staple food for a large number of people in Africa and Asia, in dry regions with low rainfall and in poor (less-fertile) soils. We may note that water availability and soil quality were the reasons farmers chose cassava and millet farming; they would have probably chosen rice or wheat cultivation if they had adequate water resources or fertile soil.

The major millets consumed across the world are pearl millet, finger millet, foxtail millet, and sorghum. Pearl millet accounts for 50% of world millet production, foxtail millet accounts for 19%, and finger millet accounts for 11%.[14] All millets have various toxins and antinutrients in them. When millets are not processed or cooked properly, the antinutrients in millets can lead to thyroid enlargement and development of goiter. As in the case of cassava, consumption of millets leads to general disruption of the bodily functions, and thyroid gland is one of them. In India, finger-millet flour is often soaked in water and fermented overnight before cooking the next morning. Thus, fermentation is the common method of reducing/eliminating goiter-causing toxins when cooking foods like cassava and finger millet.

Vegetables

Vegetables like cabbage, kale, cauliflower, and broccoli contain antithyroid substances,[10] which block the use of iodine by the thyroid gland and cause goiter. However, we consume these vegetables occasionally (and not as staple food). Also, proper cooking significantly reduces the goiter-causing effect of these vegetables. For example, cabbage is usually fermented or cooked (boiled) thoroughly. When in doubt, the traditional cooking method is the ideal choice to mitigate the goiter-causing propensity of foods.

Soyabean and Peanuts

Soyabean and peanuts (groundnuts) are two widely consumed foods that have significant goiter-causing properties. In experiments with rats, McCarrison showed that 33% of the rats developed goiter when fed on a diet of soyabeans or peanuts as the sole source of vitamins.[15] The mean thyroid gland weight in rats fed a synthetic diet with soyabeans as the sole source of vitamins was 21 grams in comparison with the 8 grams in rats fed a perfectly constituted diet consisting of freshly ground whole-wheat flour, milk, butter, sprouted legume, root vegetables, green leafy vegetables, water, and occasionally fresh meat. None of the rats on the perfectly constituted diet developed goiter. Similarly, the mean thyroid gland weight in rats fed on a synthetic diet with peanuts as the sole source of vitamins was 17 grams.

To mitigate goiter-causing properties of peanuts, peanuts were traditionally roasted or boiled. Fermentation is the common process used for processing soyabeans in many Chinese, Japanese and Korean dishes.

Table 7.1 Magnesium and potassium content in various staple foods (in 100 grams dry weight)[24]

Staple food	Magnesium	Potassium	Potassium to Magnesium Ratio
Potato	110 mg	2005 mg	18.2
Sweet Potato	109 mg	1465 mg	13.4
Cassava	53 mg	678 mg	12.8
Soyabeans, green	203 mg	1938 mg	9.5
Rice	28 mg	131 mg	4.7
Wheat	145 mg	417 mg	2.9

Table 7.1 shows magnesium and potassium content in various staple foods and the ratio of potassium to magnesium in these staple foods. Rather than the absolute amount of potassium, the ratio of potassium to magnesium is important in the context of thyroid disease. It may be noted that potassium to magnesium ratio is exceedingly high in all the thyroid-disease-causing foods. For example, the potassium to magnesium ratio of sweet potato is four and a half times that of wheat. The potassium to magnesium ratio of cassava is about four times that of wheat and two and a half times that of rice. The traditional thyroid disease theory focuses on goiter-causing substances in sweet potato and cassava. However, the imbalance in electrolytes in these staple foods may be the actual reason why these staple foods may be causing thyroid disease. As in the case of limestone-source water, these staple foods when consumed may be causing imbalance in the blood of man

because of the imbalance in the electrolytes in these staple foods. The same reasoning may be extended to other foods that are known to cause thyroid disease.

Milk

Milk is a food consumed all over the world. But milk can be goiter-causing.

In southern Tasmania, Australia, an annual epidemic of goiter occurred among children attending three schools.[4] It was noted that the same children were affected each year, about 30% of the students. No differences were found in the physical environment, economic status, way of life, dietary pattern, or milk consumption of the children who had a normal thyroid gland and those who had a regularly enlarged thyroid. The seasonal increase in size coincided with the spring flush of pastures and weeds, which supported the hypothesis that a food goitrogen originating in pastures and present in the milk was responsible for the goiter epidemics.[4] There was some evidence that susceptibility to the food goitrogen was an inherent characteristic of the children affected. As we have seen in the chapter on soil, spring herbage in few cases has a detrimental effect on the health of the animal. The above observation in Australia confirms that herbage affects human beings through milk.

In Finland too, the cause of goiter in an endemic goiter region was attributed to milk.[16] The reason milk caused goiter was attributed to the presence of a goitrin (thioglycoside) present in the milk. The source of this goitrin was the grass and weeds on which the cows grazed.

Soyabean meal, which is commonly used as cattle-feed in many countries, is a goitrogen.[17] Soyabean meal prevents normal reabsorption of iodine from the intestines, which results in larger loses of iodine in feces than normal. The milk of cows feeding on soyabean meal is likely goitrogenic too.

Thiocyanate is another goitrogen factor in herbage. Thiocyanate is a goiter-producing factor because it impedes the utilization of iodine in the blood by the thyroid gland. It was shown that in sheep consuming ordinary white clover, the thiocyanate in the blood was 2.2 mg of in 100 ml of blood.[2(p79)] In sheep consuming selected white clover, the thiocyanate in their blood was 8.3 mg of thiocyanate in 100 ml of blood, i.e., four times as much.[2(p79)] The selected white clover variety has, on an average, 14 times higher iodine content than normal white clover,[2(p80)] but despite the high iodine content, it was causing goiter because of the goitrogenic substance in it. While the ordinary clover variety has a lower iodine content, it did not cause thyroid disease. This shows that the iodine content of a food item is not important in the cause of thyroid disease; what is important is the goitrogenic content of the food item. The milk of cattle consuming such goitrogenic clover/feed is likely to be goitrogenic.

In my native village in India, I made similar observations. The milk of native-breed cows grazing exclusively on grass and shrubs growing on limestone soil was goitrogenic, especially during the winter season. On the other hand, the milk of high-yielding jersey-breed cows feeding on dry hay of paddy, grass, and assorted shrubs was not goitrogenic. This is contrary to what one would have expected.

Generally, native-breed cow milk has A2 protein, which is considered relatively healthy. Yet, in the context of thyroid disease, this observation shows that feed has a bigger role on the quality of the milk than the genetic variety of the cow.

The reasoning that milk causes goiter because of goiter-causing substances in the herbage is the traditional theory. It is possible that the goiter-causing propensity of milk may be because of the electrolyte-imbalance-causing property of the specific herbage discussed.

In summary, certain foods and goiter-causing substances in them or electrolyte-imbalance-causing properties in them, can cause goiter or hypothyroidism symptoms in man. These foods may be causing goiter or thyroid disease by ultimately increasing the blood plasma pH, which as we have seen previously is the immediate cause of hypothyroidism symptoms.

ii. Influence of Thyroid Gland on Metabolism of Food

Until now, we have seen the influence of various foods on the thyroid gland. Now, we will see the influence of thyroid gland on food metabolism.

Thyroid Hormones and Metabolism of Food

The food we eat is digested in the stomach and small intestine. The blood then takes the digested food to each cell in the body. Inside each cell, the digested food is turned into energy. A little thyroid hormone is used in each cell in the process of turning food into energy. The thyroid hormones act directly on the mitochondria[18(p347)] (the energy making organ in the cell). Without the thyroid hormone, this process of making energy is disrupted. In hypothyroidism, because of the low thyroid hormone, less energy is produced in the cells, resulting in fatigue. In hypothyroidism, because of the low thyroid hormone and low energy production, there is less heat generated, resulting in the cold-feeling/cold-temperature of the body.

Thyroid Hormones and Carbohydrates, Proteins, and Fats Influence Each Other

Thyroid hormones control carbohydrate, protein, and fat metabolism, i.e., making and breakdown of carbohydrates, proteins, and fats. Both a deficiency and an excess thyroid hormone are harmful to the making of carbohydrates, proteins, and fats.[18(p353–354)] For example, when people with normal thyroid function are treated with thyroid hormone medication, it results in decreased protein synthesis, while in hypothyroid patients, the same dose increases protein synthesis to normal levels.[18(p354)] Also, rats and men synthesize cholesterol more rapidly than normal when given thyroid hormone; hence, there is low cholesterol when excess thyroid hormone is supplied.[18(p354)]

Carbohydrates from the food we eat is turned into glucose. Glucose is used in the cells for making energy, and some of it is stored in liver and muscles in the form of glycogen. Thyroid hormones control the rates of glycogen synthesis and breakdown. The glycogen contents of liver and muscle are markedly diminished in hyperthyroid patients.[19] As a corollary, it follows that there must be excess glycogen in the liver and muscle in hypothyroidism, resulting in the key symptoms of hypothyroidism, i.e., bloated body and flabby skin.

Thyroid Hormones and Vitamins Influence Each Other

Thyroid hormones control the utilization and synthesis of B vitamins, vitamin C and fat-soluble vitamins such as vitamin A.[18(p356)] Vitamins B1, B5, B6, B12 and C have been found to be low in hyperthyroid/thyrotoxic patients.[18(p356)] Vitamin A synthesis requires thyroid hormone.[18(p356)] Both hypothyroid and hyperthyroid patients have poor adaption to darkness,[20] which is a key sign of night blindness, and night blindness is caused by vitamin A deficiency. This shows the interrelationship between thyroid hormones and vitamins.

Thyroid Hormones and Minerals Influence Each Other

Thyroid hormones and calcium, magnesium, and phosphorous metabolism influence each other. For example, magnesium metabolism depends on thyroid status and the thyroid status depends on magnesium.[18(p357)] Plasma magnesium is low in hyperthyroidism and high in hypothyroidism.[18(p357)]

Selenium and Thyroid Hormones

Although a mineral, selenium needs special mention because of its importance in the context of thyroid gland. Selenium concentration is higher in the thyroid gland than in any other organ in the body. Like iodine, selenium plays an important role in thyroid hormone synthesis (making) and metabolism.[21] Selenium is required for the conversion of the T_4 form of the thyroid hormone into the more active T_3 form. However, selenium deficiency does not get much attention in thyroid disease. Iodine gets all the attention, so much so that iodine deficiency is considered as the cause of thyroid disease.

Epidemiological evidence (the study of the distribution, patterns and determinants of health and disease in a defined population) supports a relationship between selenium levels and thyroid gland function. There is an inverse relationship between blood selenium concentrations and thyroid volume, goiter risk, and thyroid tissue damage risk.[22] A study of adults with mild iodine deficiency in Denmark found a significant inverse association between serum selenium concentration and thyroid volume in women,[23] i.e., lower the selenium, the more enlarged was the thyroid gland.

In summary, we may say that the thyroid gland influences the metabolism of carbohydrates, proteins, fats, vitamins, and minerals. The thyroid gland is in turn influenced by all these substances. Deficiencies or excesses of any of these substances has an impact on the thyroid gland. Each of these substances is required in the right amount, neither less nor more. Similarly, deficient or excess thyroid hormone secretion has an impact on each of these substances. Thus, the thyroid gland and food influence each other. The implication of these findings is that we need to ensure variety and moderation in the foods we consume.

Is the Cause of Thyroid Disease Food or Water?

Through most of this book, I have shown that drinking water from a limestone source is the primary cause of thyroid disease. This conclusion still stands. No one in the United States eats millets, cassava or soy as a staple food. Yet, thyroid disease is rampant in United States. Other goitrogenic foods like cabbage and broccoli are eaten in the United States, but they are not staple foods. Milk from soyabean-meal-fed cows may be a source of goiter-causing substance in the United States. But, overall, although food is a likely cause of thyroid disease, it is not the primary cause. Water is still the primary source of thyroid disease.

References

1. McCarrison R. *The Thyroid Gland in Health and Disease*. New York: William Wood & Co.; 1917.

2. Voisin A. New strains of white clover which cause bloat and affect the thyroid gland. In: *Soil, Grass and Cancer*. London: Crosby Lockwood & Son; 1959.

3. Scott H, Gupta SP. The distribution of goitre in the United Provinces. *Ind Jour Med Res.* 1934;XXI(3):649-654.

4. Clements FW, Health significance of endemic goitre and related conditions. In: *Endemic Goitre.* Monograph Series No.44. Geneva: World Health Organization; 1960:239.

5. Howeler R, Lutaladio N, Thomas G. Save and grow cassava. Rome: Food and Agriculture Organization. 2013. In: Cassava. Wikipedia. https://en.wikipedia.org/wiki/Cassava. Accessed May 8, 2022.

6. Bolarinwa IF, Oke MO, Olaniyan SA, and Ajala AS. A review of cyanogenic glycosides in edible plants. In: Soloneski S, Larramendy ML, eds. *Toxicology—New Aspects to This Scientific Conundrum.* https://www.intechopen.com/chapters/52207. Updated October 26, 2016. Accessed May 8, 2022..

7. Cereda MP, Mattos MCY. Linamarin: The toxic compound of cassava. *J Venom Animals and Toxins.* 1996;2:6-12.

8. Gomez G, Valdivieso M. The effect of variety and plant age on cyanide content, chemical composition and quality of cassava roots. *Nutr Rep Int.*1983;27(4):857-865.

9. Wagner H. Cassava's cyanide-producing abilities can cause neuropathy. In: Cassava. Wikipedia. https://en.wikipedia.org/wiki/Cassava. Archived from the original on September 24, 2010. Accessed May 8, 2022.

10. Siritunga D, Sayre RT. Transgenic approaches for cyanogen reduction in cassava. *J AOAC Int.* 2007;90(5):1450-1455. In: Cassava. Wikipedia. https://en.wikipedia.org/wiki/Cassava. Accessed May 8,2022.

11. Akindahunsi AA, Grissom FE, Adewusi SR, Afolabi OA, Torimiro SE, Oke OL. Parameters of thyroid function in the endemic goitre of Akungba and Oke-Agbe villages of Akoko area of southwestern Nigeria. *African J Med Medical Sci.*1998:27(3/4): 239-242

In: Cassava. Wikipedia. https://en.wikipedia.org/wiki/Cassava. Accessed May 8,2022.

12. Bumoko GM, Sadiki NH, Rwatambuga A, et al. Lower serum levels of selenium, copper, and zinc are related to neuromotor impairments in children with konzo. *J Neurol Sci.* 2015;349 (1/2): 149-153 In: Cassava. Wikipedia. https://en.wikipedia.org/wiki/Cassava. Accessed May 8,2022.
13. Oboh G, Oladunmoye MK. Biochemical changes in micro-fungi fermented cassava flour produced from low- and medium-cyanide variety of cassava tubers. *Nutr Health.*2007;18 (4): 355-367 In: Cassava. Wikipedia. https://en.wikipedia.org/wiki/Cassava. Accessed May 8,2022.
14. Taylor JRN. Millets: Their unique nutritional and health-promoting attributes. In: *Gluten-Free Ancient Grains.* Woodhead Publishing Series in Food Science, Technology and Nutrition; 2017:55-103.
15. McCarrison R. A paper on food and goitre. *Brit Med J.* Oct.14,1933;672.
16. Gaitan E. Goitrogens in the etiology of endemic goiter. In: Stanbury JB, Hetzel BS, eds. *Endemic Goiter and Endemic Cretinism.* John Wiley; 1980:227.
17. Hemken RW, Vandersall JH, Sass BA, Hibbs JW. Goitrogenic effects of a corn silage-soyabean meal supplemented ration. *J Dairy Sci.*1970;54(1):85-88.
18. Hoch FL. Biochemistry of hyperthyroidism and hypothyroidism. *Postgrad Med J.* 1968;44:347-362.
19. Chilson OP, Sacks J. Effect of hyperthyroidism on distribution of adenosine phosphates and glycogen in liver. *Proc Soc Exp Biol.*1959;101(2):331-332 In: Hoch FL. Biochemistry of Hyperthyroidism and Hypothyroidism. *Postgrad. Med. J.* May 1968;44:354.

20. Wohl MG, Feldman JB. Vitamin A deficiency in disease of the thyroid gland: Its detection by dark adaption. *Endocrinology.* 1939; 24:389 In: Hoch FL. Biochemistry of Hyperthyroidism and Hypothyroidism. *Postgrad. Med. J.* May 1968;44:356.

21. Selenium factsheet for health professionals. National Institutes of Health. https://ods.od.nih.gov/factsheets/Selenium-HealthProfessional/. Updated March 26, 2021. Accessed May 8, 2022.

22. Derumeaux H, Valeix P, Castetbon K, et al. Association of selenium with thyroid volume and echo structure in 35- to 60-year-old French adults. *Eur J Endocrinol.* 2003;148(3):309-315. In: Selenium Factsheet for Health Professionals. National Institutes of Health. https://ods.od.nih.gov/factsheets/Selenium-HealthProfessional/. Updated March 26,2021. Accessed May 8,2022.

23. Rasmussen LB, Schomburg L, Kohrle J, et al. Selenium status, thyroid volume, and multiple nodule formation in an area with mild iodine deficiency. *Eur J Endocrinol.* 2011;164:585-90. In: Selenium Factsheet for Health Professionals. National Institutes of Health. https://ods.od.nih.gov/factsheets/Selenium-HealthProfessional/. Updated March 26,2021. Accessed May 8,2022.

24. Potato. Wikipedia. https://en.wikipedia.org/wiki/Potato. Accessed September 23, 2022.

Chapter 8

Thyroid Gland—A Few Insights

i. Thyroid Gland Function Fluctuates Even in Healthy People

Even in healthy people, the functioning of thyroid gland fluctuates, depending on factors like stage of life, season, place of residence, age, and sex.

Stage of Life—Puberty, Pregnancy, Lactation

In endemic areas, among girls, the highest incidence of goiter was at the age of puberty (12–18 years).[1(p235)] It usually appeared 2–3 years before or after commencement of menstruation.[2(p27)] But then, it sometimes disappeared spontaneously when menstruation went on in a regular manner. Among boys, the peak of goiter was also at the time of puberty (9 to 13 years).[1(p235),2(p28)]

What is so unique about puberty? Puberty is the time when physical growth of the body reaches its peak, and both bone and muscle growth are at their peak toward the end of puberty. The maximum height of an individual is reached toward the end of puberty; one usually does not grow in height after puberty. Another significant change during puberty is that the body is prepared for sexual life. Both physical growth and sexual development during puberty put an additional burden on the thyroid gland. When the thyroid gland is not able to fulfill the additional demand put on it, it results in goiter.

Goiter usually subsided after puberty even in endemic areas. As goiter appeared the most during the menstruation and sexual development phase of puberty, it would appear there is some connection between the uterus and the thyroid gland.[2(p29)] It is also possible that blood is relatively more alkaline during puberty, during the physical growth and sexual development phases, and this increase in alkalinity may be the cause of the enlargement of thyroid gland/goiter.

Table 8.1 Age-wise incidence of goiter in the private practice of Dr. Paley, England, 1830–38

Age 1–11		Age 12–19		Age 20–62	
Age	**Number of cases**	**Age**	**Number of cases**	**Age**	**Number of cases**
1	0	12	3	20	8
2	0	13	3	21	3
3	0	14	11	22	5
4	2	15	6	23	3
5	2	16	3	24	2
6	0	17	13	25	2
7	3	18	8	26	1
8	1	19	6	28	2
9	1			29	2
10	2			30	5
11	2			31	1
				34	1
				36	1
				40	2
				42, 44, 45, 46, 50, 60, & 62 each	1
Total	**13**		**53**		**45**

Table 8.1 shows the age-wise incidence of goiter, as noted by Dr. Pale of England, in a nine-year period between 1830 and 1838.[2(p36)]

We may infer from Table 8.1 that goiter was relatively rare before age 10 and after age 40. The highest incidence was between the ages 14–20. Out of 101 cases, 95 were female and 6 were male.

Table 8.2 Age-wise onset of hypothyroidism (myxedema) as noted by George Murray, Professor of Comparative Pathology in the University of Durham, about the year 1900.

Age between (years)	Males	Females	Total
15 and 20	1	8	9
20 and 25	1	22	23
25 and 30	4	21	25
30 and 35	0	32	32
35 and 40	8	46	54
40 and 45	7	52	59
45 and 50	6	35	41
50 and 55	4	25	29
55 and 60	2	26	28
60 and 70	0	10	10
70 and 80	1	1	2
Total	**34**	**278**	**312**

Table 8.2 shows the age-wise incidence of hypothyroidism (myxoedema was the name used for hypothyroidism in the past) about the year 1900, in the practice of George Murray, who was Professor of Comparative Pathology at the University of Durham and Physician to the Royal Infirmary, Newcastle.[35]

Table 8.2 was compiled from 312 cases; the table shows the age at which the symptoms were first noticed. Only cases after age 15 were recorded.

From this table, it is evident that in women, hypothyroidism (myxoedema) may develop at any time of life from age 15 to 70. From age 15 to 45, there is an increasing number of cases in each succeeding period of five years, after which the numbers diminish. More than half of the cases occured between age 30 and 50.

On comparing different periods, we find that hypothyroidism develops frequently between age 35 and 45, and more frequently during the five years following 40th year than in the five years preceding it. Thus, it is evident that between age 35 and 45, and especially during the latter half of this period, a woman is more liable to suffer from hypothyroidism (myxedema) than at any other time of her life.

It may also be noted that hypothyroidism (myxoedema) occurs nearly eight times as frequently in women as in men.

Is the cause of thyroid disease a specific life-stage or limestone-source water?

Thyroid gland enlargement at puberty is a sign of insufficient thyroid hormone synthesis for the needs of the specific life-stage.[1(p236),3] Similarly, during menstruation, pregnancy, and lactation, there is additional demand put on the thyroid gland in women. When the thyroid gland is unable to meet the additional requirements of the body during these life-stages, it results in goiter, especially when an environmental factor such as limestone-source water is present. It is also possible that these life-stages are associated with increased alkalinity of the blood, and the additional alkalinity caused by limestone-source water may be causing thyroid gland enlargement.

Life History of the Thyroid Gland[4(p27–31)]

The thyroid gland is one of the first endocrine glands to be formed in the womb of the mother. It becomes active by the sixth month of pregnancy. It is then involved in the development of the other organs. During the embryonic period, the developing thyroid gland is susceptible to influences that impair the mother's thyroid gland. It responds to these influences by undergoing enlargement, and sometimes succumbs by undergoing cell-death. It is these influences which determine (in the fetus) the future capacity of the child's thyroid gland. Thus, it is important to exclude all influences which depress or unduly strain the maternal thyroid gland. For this reason, it is of great importance to inquire into the prebirth history of all backward children and to examine the mother for any thyroid defect.

With the cessation of suckling, and with the commencement of taking solid food, the thyroid apparatus of the child begins to act for itself, responding to increasing growth and maturation of bodily functions.

The puberty life-stage has been discussed.

In both sexes, the sexual act increases the thyroid gland's activity, and it is liable to swell in consequence, a fact well known to primitive races. World War I brought to light the interesting fact that married men under 40 years of age were on the whole of better physique than unmarried men, a fact that was probably dependent in considerable measure on the maintenance of thyroidal activity, which marriage/sexual activity ensured. In women, marriage and childbearing conferred benefits which are due to, among other causes, the maintenance of healthy thyroid activity.

During pregnancy, the thyroid as well as the parathyroid glands are in a state of active secretion, which gradually diminishes throughout lactation. The maintenance of this state of activity is necessary for the speeding up of the mammary glands and the continued secretion of milk. Throughout the childbearing period of life, the thyroid maintains a high level of activity, reverting between successive pregnancies and lactation periods to the resting state. Examination of many pregnant women at the Queen Charlotte Hospital, London, found that about 50% showed slight thyroid swellings, which had originated during pregnancy. The gland is most likely to enlarge during the fifth and sixth month of pregnancy.

With the onset of menopause, the thyroid function becomes depressed. At this time, symptoms of hypothyroidism are apt to appear.

After age 40, the increasing years bring to the thyroid the changes incidental to advancing life. The thyroid arteries become thickened and less elastic, its connective tissue increases in amount, small cysts may arise in consequence, or calcareous deposits may occur. The thyroid epithelium becomes less active, and the colloid substance and iodine content decrease. In short, the gland undergoes a process of gradual decline. But with diminishing vital functions, the thyroid gland ceases to be of the same importance. *As the fire of life dies down, the stimulating draught of the thyroid becomes more gentle.*

In summary, it is natural for the thyroid gland function to fluctuate with life-stage and finally diminish with age. Then, how appropriate is it to artificially stimulate the thyroid gland using thyroid medication after a certain age? Two Americans, Virginia Leitner, at the age of 104, and Ernie Allison, at age of 103, were on synthetic thyroid medication for low thyroid.[5,6] If the thyroid gland is to the human body what the draught is to the fire, adding draught to fire at such an age may mean going against nature and the natural laws of life.

Season

"New goiters arise, and old goiters enlarge in the winter season." This was an observation made by Scott and Gupta in their research in 1933 at the foothills of the Himalayan Mountain range in India. This has been my personal observation too. I noticed at my residence in Visakhapatnam, my hometown, that water has more chalk (lime) from November to February, the winter months in India. During this time, a thick chalk coat forms on utensils used for boiling water and cooking. The water is not so chalky for rest of the year. Why should this be so? Limestone (calcium carbonate) has an unusual characteristic called retrograde solubility. This means that limestone becomes more soluble in water as the temperature drops.[7] Therefore, in winter, limestone in earth becomes more soluble. There is more limestone in the drinking water taken from wells and borewells.

Also, in winter season, the cold weather may reduce the body temperature, and thus increase the blood plasma pH, as temperature and pH share an inverse relationship.

Further, it was observed that the iodine content of animals investigated varied with the season of the year; it may be presumed that it does so in man.[4(p30)] The thyroid gland's activity varies with its iodine-content; the activity is at its lowest ebb during the first four months of the year. The phosphorous content also varies at the same time, in the inverse ratio to the iodine. Therefore, there are many changes related to the thyroid gland that happen with the season.

Place of Residence—Seacoast vs. Inland

We discussed this topic briefly in an earlier chapter. The average weight of the thyroid gland in adults is 36–50 grams in inland and hilly areas, whereas it is 20–30 grams near seacoast areas.[4(p4)] That is, the thyroid gland is half the weight in residents near the sea in comparison with its weight in inland residents. The lower weight of the thyroid gland near the sea may not merely mean lower functionality of the thyroid gland; it may also mean a more diseased state. Near the seacoast, there is excess salt (sodium chloride). The excess of these two electrolytes may cause acid–base imbalance in the blood and ultimately lead to a reduction in the size of the thyroid gland. This observation confirms the hypothesis that electrolytes, the strong ion difference, and the acid–base imbalance are involved in the cause of thyroid disease.

People suffering from hyperthyroidism do less well near the sea than inland. Sheep pastured near the sea show twice the amount of iodine in their thyroids than that in sheep raised inland. Excess iodine—like deficient iodine—is harmful.

Place of Residence—Altitude

There is less oxygen at higher altitudes. As oxygen is involved in metabolism within the cell, the body adjusts to this less oxygen environment through various balancing mechanisms. The functional activity of the thyroid gland appears to increase with increasing altitude of residence.[4(p30)] This increased action is necessitated by the body's need to maintain red blood cells and hemoglobin at a level appropriate to the altitude.

The presence of the bicarbonate buffer system allows for people to travel and live at high altitudes. When the partial pressure of oxygen and carbon dioxide change at high altitudes, the bicarbonate buffer system adjusts to regulate carbon dioxide while maintaining the correct pH in the body.[8] High altitude may worsen preexisting thyroid disease; because in thyroid disease, the bicarbonate buffer system is already burdened. But high altitude in itself does not cause thyroid disease.

In Peru, a high-altitude country, the higher altitude did not cause an increase in goiter rates. In Peru, moving from the coast to an ascent of the Cordillera Mountains, one encountered cases of goiter first at 250–850 metres above sea-level; at an elevation of 1000–3000 metres, the frequency increased, attaining average rates of 15%–25% and above. At this level, the disease was characterized by the presence of cretinism, myxedema, and a general state of low metabolism extending also to domestic animals.[9] At an even greater height, over 3300 metres, the goiter rate diminished, until it receded to an almost insignificant figure in places of the highest altitude. In the highest altitude, cretins and cases of myxedema were rarely seen, and it was difficult to find any animals with thyroid enlargement. Similar observations on the relationship between altitude and goiter and cretinism were noted in the Alps Mountain range in Switzerland. Thus, goiter and cretinism rates increased with increase in altitude, then decreased with increasing altitude, and at the highest altitude, goiter and cretinism did not exist.

Sex

The thyroid gland is about 33% heavier in women than in men.[4(p4)] A heavier thyroid in women shows that thyroid has a more important role to play in women than in men. As women go through more life-stages such as puberty, menstruation, pregnancy, lactation, and menopause, it is likely that the larger thyroid meets the additional demand put on it by each of these life-stages. When the thyroid is not able to meet the additional demands by the body during these life-stages, it results in thyroid disease. This is likely the reason why thyroid disease is more common in women than in men. Similarly, the thyroid gland has more iodine in adult women than in adult men. In animals too, female animals have more thyroid tissue and more iodine per unit body weight than do male animals.

Age

The size of the thyroid gland varies with age. In proportion to body weight, the thyroid gland is twice as large in infants than in adults. It forms about 1/800th part of the body weight in infants and 1/1800th part of the body weight in adults.[4(p4)] This shows that the thyroid gland may have a more important role in infants than in adults. Thyroid gland has an important role in *growth.* Growth is more important for an infant than for an adult. This probably accounts for the relatively larger size of the gland in infants than in adults. The iodine content in the thyroid gland similarly varies with age.

Confinement

There are few animals that live their lives in cages whose thyroids are wholly normal.[4(p40)] There are few fish that live their lives in tanks under artificial conditions whose thyroids are wholly normal. It follows that there will be few human beings living in confined homes and offices in whom the gland will be wholly normal.

In microscopic examination of tissues and cells of the thyroid gland, the widest variations were seen in laboratory animals confined in cages and in birds and animals in zoological gardens.[4(p40)] Domestic animals also exhibited these wide variations. Derangements of the thyroid were common, especially in fowls, affecting their egg-producing capacity. In dogs living in association with man, thyroid enlargement is almost the rule. David Marine found this abnormality in 90% of the dogs in Cleveland, USA. In animals living in the wild state, the disease was uncommon. Among fish, birds, and animals living in the wild state, away from man and civilization, wholly normal thyroids were the norm.

In confinement, there is reduced availability of oxygen. Deficient oxygen tends to increase the activity of thyroid at first and later depresses it.

Stress

Fear, anxiety, and mental stress are factors that have a great influence on the thyroid gland.[4(p59)] These mental states are an expression of fear. In the words of Crile, "Under the influence of fear, most of the organs of the body are divided sharply into two classes. First, those that are stimulated and those that are inhibited. Those that are stimulated are the entire muscular system, the vasomotor, and locomotor system, the senses of perception, the respiration, the mechanism for the erection of the hair, the sweat glands, the thyroid gland, the adrenal gland, and the special senses. On the other hand, all the digestive and procreative functions are inhibited. What is the significance of this stimulation of some and inhibition of other organs? As far as we know, the stimulated organs increase the efficiency of the animal for fight or flight."[4(p59)]

Fear may influence the thyroid gland not only directly, but indirectly through adrenal glands. Both thyroid and adrenal glands are known to be intimately associated in their activities, one stimulating the other.[4(p60)] In circumstances of fear, the adrenal glands, through the splanchnic nerves, cause the adrenalin hormone to be poured into the blood in large amounts. This may produce the staring eye, the frightened faces, the greatly increased supply of blood to the heart, lungs, brain, and muscles, the heightened activity of the thyroid, and general excitability of the sympathetic system. All these are symptoms of hyperthyroidism (Graves' disease), which has been linked to "continuous fear."

The stimulus of fear, in whatever form it may act, such as fright, constant worry, anxiety, or grief, may impose an added strain on the resources of the thyroid gland. Mental fatigue, overwork, shock of trauma, and accidents frequently trigger latent thyroid instability, precipitating the onset of thyroidal disorder.

In summary, the function of the thyroid gland varies widely, even in healthy people, with stage of life, place of residence, sex, age, confinement, and stress levels.

ii. Thyroid Gland—Physical Structure and Functions

It may seem too late in the book for a brief introduction to the thyroid gland, but it isn't. Note that we did not have to know any of the functions of thyroid gland for identifying *the cause* of thyroid disease; we solely depended on the symptoms to guide us. We will now briefly discuss the thyroid gland, its physical structure, and its functions so that we can relate its functions to other glands.

The thyroid gland is located in the front of the neck, just below the Adam's apple. Adam's apple is the small protrusion in the neck. The thyroid gland consists of two adjacent lobes (portions) of reddish-brown color, joined together by an isthmus (bridge). The thyroid gland is not merely a piece of flesh. Within the thyroid gland, there is a huge network of blood vessels (arteries and veins), a network of the lymphatic system, and a network of nerves.

The thyroid gland has one of the largest supplies of blood, relative to its size. The entire blood in the body flows through the thyroid gland every one hour. In proportion to its size, the thyroid gland receives more than five times as much blood as the kidneys.[4(p5)] We know that kidneys purify the blood; hence, all the blood must pass through the kidneys. But what relationship does the thyroid have with blood that such a large quantity should pass through it? The thyroid gland supplies thyroid hormones to the blood passing through it, which is then carried to every cell of the body.

Lymph (from Latin, meaning *water*) is a colorless, watery liquid that flows through the lymphatic system.[10] Lymph and the lymphatic system are part of the immune system. Lymph collects waste and cellular debris from interstitial fluids and returns them to the blood. Bacteria are also picked up by lymph and are destroyed in the lymph nodes. Lymph flows freely and extensively through the thyroid gland.[4(p4)] This shows a relationship between the thyroid gland and the immune system.

The thyroid gland has a good nerve supply, and both the sympathetic and parasympathetic nervous systems are connected to the thyroid gland. In experimental stimulation of nerves, the secretion of thyroid hormone starts within 5 seconds. When the phrenic nerve is joined to the peripheral portion of the cervical sympathetic in the cat, the thyroid is continuously stimulated as the animal breathes, which results in tachycardia (irregular heartbeat), increased excitability, loose motions, exophthalmos (bulging eyes), great increase in the metabolism, and in few cases, an increase in size of the adrenal glands. These are all symptoms of hyperthyroidism. In short, the nervous system stimulates the thyroid gland.

When we look at the thyroid gland under a microscope,[11] the tissue of the thyroid gland looks as in Figure 8.1.

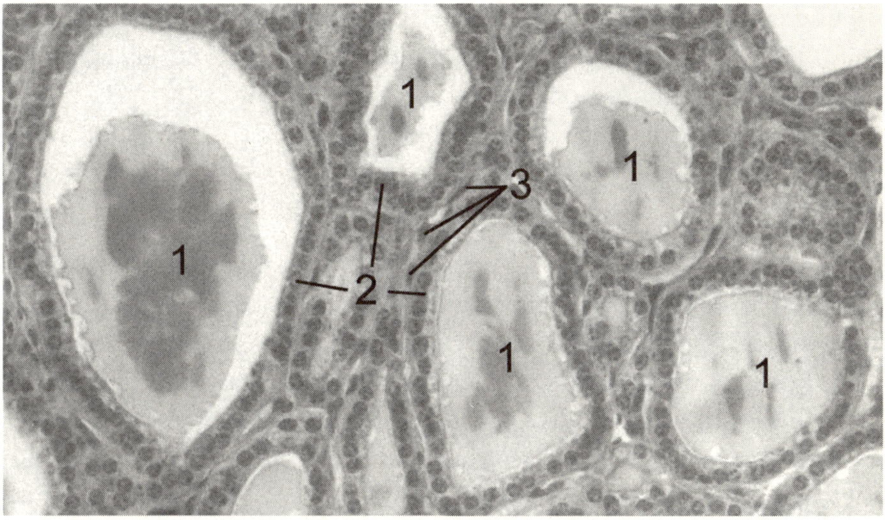

Figure 8.1 Thyroid gland tissue as seen under the microscope. 1. Colloid substance; 2. Follicular cells; 3. Endothelial cells. (Credit: Uwe Gille)

The colloid substance (#1 in the figure) forms more than half of the volume of the thyroid gland. The colloid substance has a protein called thyroglobulin, which is used to make the thyroid hormones. It also contains sodium chloride (common salt) in abundance, phosphorus, sulfur, arsenic, bromine, selenium, and iodine.[12,13] The most important constituent of the colloid substance is iodine.

The follicular cells (#2 in the figure), which are arranged in the form of a necklace, secrete the thyroid hormones triiodothyronine (T_3) and thyroxine (T_4). The follicular cells do this by transporting and metabolizing the thyroglobulin protein contained in the colloid substance, iodine and, tyrosine (an amino acid).[14] The follicular cell, along with colloid substance, is called a follicle.

In the space between the follicles are parafollicular cells (#3 in the figure). These cells secrete another thyroid hormone called calcitonin.

Thus, the thyroid gland secretes three hormones—T_3, T_4, and calcitonin. T_3 is so named because it contains three atoms of iodine per molecule and T_4 contains four atoms of iodine per molecule.[15]

To understand the function of the thyroid gland, we need to understand the function of the hormones it secretes. In the thyroid gland, about 80%–90% of the hormones produced are T_4 and 10%–20% of the hormones produced are T_3.[16,17] The function of both T_4 and T_3 hormones is similar. In a single word, the primary function of thyroid hormones is *metabolism*. As noted earlier, *the thyroid gland is to the human body what draught is to the fire.*

Once thyroid hormones are made in the thyroid gland, they are transported through blood to all cells in the body—heart cells, muscle cells, bone cells, brain cells, nerve cells, skin cells, hair cells, and so on. Once inside these cells, thyroid hormones increase the metabolism of each of these cells. That is, thyroid hormones produce energy within each of these cells. Thyroid hormones govern *the growth* of all cells and sustain their functional activity.

When a low quantity of thyroid hormones is produced by the thyroid gland, the metabolism of all the cells slows down. There is deficient consumption of oxygen. There is reduced energy. The body (heart, muscles, bones, skin, hair) becomes sluggish. The mind (brain, nerves) becomes sluggish. The result is the symptoms that we see in hypothyroidism. The low energy produced leads to low heat production, which causes the typical symptom of feeling cold in hypothyroidism.

When an excess quantity of thyroid hormone is produced by thyroid gland, the metabolism of all the cells increases. There is excess consumption of oxygen. The heart, muscles, brain, and other tissues operate at a much faster rate than normal. There is racing and irregular heartbeat, the mind is agitated, the skin becomes supple and moist, and so on. These are all symptoms of hyperthyroidism disease.

How do we know what the functions of the thyroid hormones are? We can know the functions if we remove the thyroid gland and see what happens.

When thyroid gland was completely removed during goiter surgery, surgeons noted severe hypothyroidism and cretinism-like symptoms in their patients during follow up.[18(p331–332)] The cretinism symptoms were closely related to symptoms seen in endemic cretinism.[14(p332)] In patients where the thyroid gland was partly removed, these symptoms were seen only partly. Thus, we can say that deficiency of thyroid hormones causes symptoms of endemic cretinism. These observations were confirmed through experiments on monkeys; the removal or destruction of thyroid gland resulted is cretinism symptoms.[14(p332)] Thus, the conclusion was arrived at that *loss of thyroid function* was the root cause of cretinism.

We have seen in Chapter 2 that the symptoms of endemic cretinism affect every cell of the body—bones, muscles, brain, sexual development, senses (hearing and speech), skin, hair, nails, and so on. Thus, thyroid hormones are involved in the metabolism of each and every cell in the body.

Another way to understand the functions of the thyroid gland is to administer thyroid hormone to someone and see the impact. Administration of thyroid hormone was sufficient to compensate for the deficiency of thyroid function, and this was of great significance for understanding the function of the thyroid gland.[14(p333)] Administration of animal thyroid gland preparations as medicine led to improvement in hypothyroidism symptoms. This confirmed that symptoms considered to be thyroid disease symptoms were in fact related to the thyroid gland. Thus, the symptoms confirmed *the functions* of the thyroid hormones.

The third thyroid hormone produced by the thyroid gland is *calcitonin*. Calcitonin regulates the *calcium metabolism* in the body. When there is too much calcium in the blood, the thyroid gland releases calcitonin to reduce the calcium level in the blood. This hormone works in tandem with the parathyroid hormones and vitamin D/sunlight.

Further, research has shown that thyroid hormones are also involved in maintaining the constituents of the blood, red blood cells, white blood cells, hemoglobin, and salts at a proper level and that thyroid hormones regulate blood pressure, maintain activity of sympathetic and parasympathetic nervous system, and stimulate other glands and organs.

iii. Thyroid Gland's Relationship with Other Glands

What we call thyroid disease—is it just a disease in the thyroid gland or are other glands involved too?

Haubold, a German scientist, noted that in the patients suffering from goiter, 79% were simultaneously suffering from disturbance of the pituitary gland, 68% from disturbance in the adrenal glands, 60% from disturbance in the hypothalamus, and 52% from liver conditions, and that appearance of goiter was merely a symptom of disturbance in these other glands and organs.[19(p202)]

Let us look at the relationship between thyroid gland and few other glands and organs.

Pituitary Gland

The pituitary gland is located in the brain. It is the size of an almond. Yet, it is considered a "master gland." It is considered a master gland because it regulates and influences the function of all other glands. The pituitary gland and the thyroid gland share a close relationship.

The pituitary gland secretes a hormone called thyroid stimulating hormone (TSH), which, as the name says, stimulates the thyroid gland to secrete thyroid hormones. As the amount of thyroid hormone in the blood decreases, more TSH hormone is secreted by the pituitary gland. Conversely, as the amount of thyroid hormone in the blood increases, less TSH hormone is secreted by the pituitary gland. Thus, the thyroid gland gets its instructions whether to produce thyroid hormone or not from its master, the pituitary gland.

Because of this close relationship, if the pituitary gland is diseased, it should get reflected in the functioning of the thyroid gland. Therefore, when we see a disease in the thyroid gland, it is possible that we are actually dealing with a disease in the pituitary gland. It is just that diagnostic tests for pituitary gland functioning are not so common as diagnostic tests for thyroid disease. What if the disease is actually in the pituitary gland?

Adrenal Glands

The adrenal glands are named after their location in the body. The adrenal glands are located above the kidneys. The term "adrenal" comes from Latin words *ad* ("near") and *renes* ("kidney"). Previously, adrenal glands were called suprarenal glands, which literally meant *supra* ("above") and *renes* ("kidney"), i.e., above the kidneys.

The adrenal glands make hormones such as adrenaline, aldosterone, and cortisol. The adrenal glands measure only 5 cm in length, 3 cm in width, and 1 cm in thickness. The combined weight of the two adrenal glands is 7–10 g, which is less than a third of the weight of the thyroid gland. It is surprising that a gland which weighs just a few grams performs a large number of important functions. Adrenal hormones are involved in important functions such as regulation of blood pressure, electrolyte balance, metabolism, immune system suppression, sex hormones production, and stress response. These are all functions that even thyroid gland is known to be involved in.

We have seen in previous chapters that thyroid disease has a basis in electrolyte imbalance produced by drinking limestone-source water. We can see from the description here that adrenal glands are also involved in maintaining electrolyte balance. When there is imbalance of electrolytes, then both the thyroid gland and the adrenal glands should become dysfunctional. What we call thyroid disease may actually be an adrenal disease also. As adrenal glands are located deep inside our body, near the kidneys, the disease in them is not easily visible, whereas the disease in thyroid gland is visible just by looking at the neck of a goitrous person. The symptoms related to adrenal gland disease may have got clubbed under thyroid disease.

The thyroid gland stimulates and is stimulated by the adrenal glands, thus indirectly controlling blood pressure, and securing the supply of oxygenated blood to all parts of the body. The absence of steroid hormones produced by the adrenal cortex bring about an increase in size of the thyroid gland.

The adrenal glands release a hormone called cortisol. The pituitary gland makes a hormone called ACTH. ACTH controls the production of cortisol. Therefore, the pituitary gland controls the adrenal gland just like it controls the thyroid gland. Administration of thyroid hormone (similar to levothyroxine/synthetic thyroid hormone tablets) to mice gives rise to intensive cortisone secretion by the adrenal glands. Thus, the functioning of adrenal glands, pituitary glands, and the thyroid gland is closely interrelated.

Pineal Gland

Rene Descartes, a French philosopher, mathematician, and scientist, called the pineal gland *the principal seat of the soul.*[20] Descartes wrote that "The body and spirit meet here, and each affects the other."[21] In Indian mysticism, the pineal gland is considered *the third eye,* an invisible eye which is the center of our intuition. Thus, both the Western and the Eastern philosophies seem to have significance attached to the pineal gland.

The pineal gland is a small endocrine gland in the brain. The shape of the gland resembles a pine cone, which gives it its name.[22] It weighs 0.1 gram (0.004 ounce) and is 0.8 cm (0.3 inches) in length, i.e., it is less than a tenth of a gram and is less than one centimeter.[23]

The pineal gland produces a hormone called melatonin. Melatonin is a darkness hormone; its production is stimulated by darkness. Light inhibits the production of melatonin hormone.

A key function of melatonin is maintaining circadian rhythm. Circadian rhythm refers to the daily, seasonal, and annual *rhythm* of the body. Melatonin hormone, through its role in circadian rhythm, plays an important role in the regulation of energy metabolism, glucose homeostasis/balance, and body temperature regulation.[24] For example, peak melatonin is associated with the lowest body temperature, maximum tiredness, lowest alertness, and performance.[25] These are all symptoms of hypothyroidism. This shows that thyroid disease symptoms are associated with peak melatonin production. Therefore, are thyroid disease symptoms due to low thyroid hormone production or excess melatonin production? In other words, are the symptoms due to disease in the thyroid gland or pineal gland?

Melatonin also plays a role in puberty, in menstrual cycle, and in reproductive function.[20] Even thyroid gland is involved in puberty, menstruation, and reproductive function. This shows the interconnectedness of the functioning of the pineal gland and the thyroid gland.

Sexual Glands

During puberty (age 11–17), the human body is prepared for sexual life. This is also when the thyroid gland is most strained. In chapter 3, we noted that goiter occurrence peaks during puberty. This shows the relationship between sexual development and thyroid hormone requirement. In cretinism, the extreme form of low thyroid disease, there is an extreme sexual drive. We also noted previously that married men under 40 years of age (i.e., men with active sexual life) were on the whole of better physique than the unmarried men, showing the relationship between sexual life and physical growth. Often, infertility is associated with low thyroid hormones. These observations show the interconnectedness of sexual glands and the thyroid gland.

Thymus Gland

Thymus is a gland located below the breastbone, a long flat bone in the center of the chest. The thymus continues to grow after birth, reaching maximum size of 40-50 grams by puberty.[26,27,28] After puberty, it decreases in size, and in old age, it typically weighs 5–15 grams. We may note that puberty is also the time when the thyroid gland is needed the most. This shows that both the thyroid gland and thymus gland operate at their peak during puberty.

The thymus gland's primarily role is protection of the body against infection. It is part of the immune system. It makes white blood cells, commonly known as T lymphocytes or T cells. T cells are named after the organ of their origin, i.e., the thymus.

As noted earlier, in hypothyroidism, there is a reduction in number of one type of white blood cells called lymphocytes, usually from 30%–18% of total white blood cells.[18] Lymphocytes fight infections by creating antibodies against bacteria, virus, and other invaders. There is also an increase in the number of another type of white blood cells called eosinophils, usually from 2%–3% to 11%–16% of white blood cells. Eosinophils are known for their role in allergy symptoms. They also fight parasites, and viral and fungal infections. Thus, the thymus gland is involved in the generation of lymphocytes, and lymphocytes are reduced in hypothyroidism. This shows the interconnectedness between the thymus gland and the thyroid gland.

Pancreas

An observation in my hometown is that people who suffer from hypothyroidism usually do not suffer from diabetes. There may be few exceptions to this general trend. On the other hand, people who suffer from hyperthyroidism often show symptoms of diabetes. The relationship between mild and transient diabetes in hyperthyroidism has been frequently described in the literature.[29]

The primarily role of thyroid hormones is metabolism. Metabolism involves two broad processes—catabolism and anabolism. Catabolism is the breakdown of large molecules into smaller ones. For example, catabolism involves breakdown of carbohydrates into glucose, fats into fatty acids, and proteins into amino acids. Catabolism releases energy and heat. Thyroid hormones are involved in catabolism.

Anabolism, on the other hand, builds complex molecules from simpler ones. Anabolism builds tissues and organs using the smaller units created by catabolism. Anabolism makes proteins (from amino acids) and fats (from fatty acids). Examples of anabolism are increase in muscle mass and building bone. While catabolism releases energy, anabolism uses energy. Insulin, the hormones released by pancreases, is involved in anabolism. Thus, thyroid hormones and insulin hormones work complementarily in the process of metabolism, although on opposite processes in metabolism.

When metabolism in the body slows, blood glucose levels drop. In hypothyroidism, when there is both hypothyroidism and diabetes in a patient, it is often necessary to reduce the dose of diabetes medicines to prevent low blood glucose.

It is the primary role of pancreas and its hormone insulin to control glucose levels in the blood. When the glucose level is high, the hormone insulin is secreted to reduce the glucose level. When the glucose level is low, the hormone glucagon is secreted to increase the glucose level. Glucagon increases the glucose level by promoting the creation of glucose and the breakdown of glycogen to glucose in the liver.[30] It also decreases the uptake of glucose in fat and muscle. Even thyroid gland is involved in the metabolism of carbohydrates and glucose. This shows that hormones of both thyroid gland and pancreas are involved in glucose metabolism.

The primary mechanism for release of insulin involves calcium. A significantly higher amount of calcium in the cell cytoplasm causes the release of previously synthesized insulin (stored in intracellular secretory vesicles) into the blood.[31] We have earlier seen the importance of calcium ions in relation to thyroid disease.

This brief discussion shows that thyroid gland and pancreas work complementarily in metabolism.

Liver

Jaundice was a common symptom in cretinism. In 1897, Henry Koplik, a physician at the Mount Sinai Hospital in New York City, described a few cases of cretinism in the United States.[32] In each of these cases, jaundice was observed at birth. The jaundice typically lasted 4–6 weeks. Jaundice is normally a sign of liver disease. In jaundice, the white of the eyes and skin turn yellow. The similar symptoms in jaundice and cretinism show the connection between thyroid gland and liver.

Between 1784 and 1789, goiter and night-blindness occurred simultaneously in the French Royal Regiment stationed at Nancy, France.[15(p205–206)] We know that night blindness is caused by vitamin A deficiency. About 80%–90% of the total body reserves of vitamin A are in the liver. This again shows that thyroid gland and liver are connected.

The liver plays an important role in the metabolism of lipids/fats. It produces bile, which is required for emulsifying fats and absorption of various fat-soluble vitamins such as vitamin A, D, E, and K.

The liver plays an important role in vitamin D metabolism. Sunlight provides vitamin D through skin. The liver converts the vitamin D received from the sun into a more usable form, 25OHD. Sunlight (vitamin D) acts as medicine in cretinism. This shows the importance of the liver in producing fat-soluble vitamin D and in thyroid health.

Fatigue is a common complaint in hypothyroidism, and it is also the most common complaint reported by patients with liver disorders.[33] Fatigue is also the key symptom in anemia, which is popularly referred to as tired blood. About 13% of the blood in the body is in the liver at any given point of time. About 1.7 liters of blood is filtered in the liver per minute. The nutrient-filled blood from intestines and stomach first enters the liver. The liver enzymes process these nutrients before sending the blood for use to the rest of the body. The liver filters the blood and removes harmful substances like toxins, drugs, and waste products. This shows the importance of the liver in maintaining the health of blood. When liver is unable to process the nutrients in the blood or clear the waste from the blood, the blood eventually gets loaded with waste products. The blood becomes tired, the individual becomes tired/fatigued, which is a key symptom in both liver disease and thyroid disease.

The liver is also involved in the regulation of pH. We have seen earlier that it is the disruption of pH balance that causes thyroid disease. Thus, the liver has a direct impact on thyroid health.

The liver is involved in the metabolism of carbohydrates, proteins, and fats. It is the primary place where proteins are metabolized, synthesized, and later degraded. The thyroid regulates the storage of glycogen and its discharge from the liver. Thus, the liver and the thyroid gland work complementarily in metabolism.

The liver filters the blood, eliminates toxins from the bloodstream, and breaks down used red blood cells. Even thyroid hormones are involved in breaking down exhausted and dead cells.

The blood proteins—albumin, globulin, and fibrinogen—are made in the liver (except for few globulin proteins). Albumin and globulin proteins are used as buffers in acid–base balance, which when deranged causes thyroid disease.

We thus see that liver and thyroid gland are inextricably linked in their functioning. If the liver is diseased, it should get reflected in the functioning of the thyroid gland, and vice versa. When someone says they have a thyroid disease, they may also be saying that they have a liver disease, or their liver function is disrupted.

Lungs and Kidneys

Lungs and kidneys act as buffers in maintaining acid–base balance in the body. It is acid–base imbalance that causes thyroid disease. Therefore, lungs and kidneys have a direct role in the health of the thyroid gland.

The lungs act as buffers by increasing or decreasing the breathing rate to make the blood plasma more alkaline or acidic, depending on the need. Lungs act within a few minutes to bring about acid–base balance.

The kidneys play a direct role in acid–base balance by increasing or decreasing reabsorption of various electrolytes (sodium, chloride, phosphate, bicarbonate, and potassium) when blood passes through them. The kidneys bring about acid–base balance more slowly than do the lungs; they take few days in bringing about acid–base balance in comparison with a few minutes taken by lungs.

In addition to acid–base balance, the kidneys control the volume of various body fluids. One of the symptoms of hypothyroidism is constipation. Constipation is passing of dry and hard stools. There is lack of water/fluid in the stools. In addition to impaired muscle contraction discussed previously as the cause of constipation, fluid imbalance may also have a role in causing constipation. Thus, the kidneys may play a role in this key symptom of hypothyroidism through their role in fluid balance.

Kidneys also secrete calcitriol hormone, an activated form of Vitamin D, which promotes intestinal absorption of calcium and the renal reabsorption of phosphate.[34] Calcium metabolism is disrupted in thyroid disease. The kidneys, through their role in calcium metabolism, may have a role in calcium/bone-related symptoms of thyroid disease.

Thus, the lungs and kidneys have a direct role in the health or disease of thyroid gland.

Parathyroid Glands

Of all the glands discussed till now, the parathyroid glands are located closest to the thyroid gland. In fact, the word *parathyroid* means *situated near the thyroid.* There are four parathyroid glands located on either side of the thyroid. Each parathyroid gland is about the size of a pea and weighs about 35–55 milligrams. The parathyroid glands are not only located close to the thyroid but are also similar in function to the thyroid.

The main function of the parathyroid glands is to maintain the body's calcium levels within a very narrow range. The parathyroid gland secretes a hormone called parathyroid hormone. This hormone is secreted when the blood calcium levels are low. The parathyroid hormone increases calcium levels in blood through its action on bones (releasing calcium from bones), kidneys (increasing absorption of calcium through kidneys), and intestine (increasing absorption of calcium through action on vitamin D).

While the parathyroid hormone acts to increase calcium level in the blood, the thyroid gland produces calcitonin to reduce the level of calcium in the blood. Thus, the parathyroid and thyroid have opposite affects depending on the calcium level in the blood.

Calcium is important in the function of bones, muscles, and nerves. In the past, when parathyroid glands were removed along with the thyroid gland during surgery, it led to tetany (severe muscle spasms), often resulting in death of the patient. Calcium is required to transmit muscle and nerve impulses, i.e., transmitting information from one muscle/nerve to the next muscle/nerve. When there is excess or deficiency of calcium, the muscle and nerve functions get disrupted. In hypothyroidism, we have many muscle and nerve symptoms. So, are these symptoms caused by defects in the thyroid gland or parathyroid glands?

Role of Various Glands, Hormones, Organs, and Minerals in Calcium Metabolism

The key symptoms of cretinism and hypothyroidism are bone-related symptoms, deformed bones, and rheumatic joint pains. But it is not just the thyroid gland which is involved in bone or calcium metabolism; there are other hormones and minerals that play a role. The health of bone and calcium metabolism is dependent on various glands (parathyroid gland, thyroid gland), hormones (parathyroid hormone, vitamin D, calcitonin), organs (skin, liver, kidneys), and minerals (magnesium, phosphate). When we see bone-related symptoms in a person, the impairment could be in any of the above.

In summary, the thyroid gland is dependent on various glands, hormones, and organs in the body for discharge of its functions. And similarly, various glands, hormones, and organs are dependent on the thyroid gland for discharge of their functions. Therefore, when we see thyroid disease symptoms in a person, the symptoms could be due to disease in any of these other glands or organs.

References

1. Clements FW, Health significance of endemic goitre and related conditions. In: *Endemic Goitre.* Monograph Series No.44. Geneva: World Health Organization; 1960:235.
2. Inglis J. *Treatise on English Bronchocele: With a Few Remarks on the Use of Iodine and Its Compounds*. London: Longman, Orme, Brown, Green, and Longmans; 1838.
3. Stott H, Bhatia BB, Lal RS, Rai KC. The distribution and cause of endemic goitre in the United Provinces. *Indian J. Med. Res.*1931;18:1059-1085.
4. McCarrison R. *The Thyroid Gland in Health and Disease*. New York: William Wood & Company; 1917.
5. Leitner V. I get asked a lot about longevity. It helps that I'm 104. https://www.statnews.com/2019/07/17/aging-longevity-centenarian-oral-history/. Accessed May 8, 2022.
6. Ernie Irene Allison. https://obituaries.mcalesternews.com/obituary/ernie-allison-1084213329. Published January 15, 2022. Accessed May 8, 2022.
7. Carbonate Rock. Wikipedia. https://en.wikipedia.org/wiki/Carbonate_rock./. Accessed May 8, 2022.
8. Transport of carbon dioxide in the blood. Lumen. https://courses.lumenlearning.com/wm-biology2/chapter/transport-of-carbon-dioxide-in-the-blood/. Accessed May 8, 2022.
9. Kelly FC, Snedden WW. Prevalence and geographical distribution of endemic goitre. In: *Endemic Goitre*. Monograph Series No.44. Geneva: World Health Organization; 1960:48.
10. Lymph. Wikipedia. https://en.wikipedia.org/wiki/Lymph. Accessed May 8, 2022.
11. Gille U. Section of a thyroid gland under the microscope. Wikipedia. https://en.wikipedia.org/wiki/Thyroid#/media/File:Thyroid-histology.jpg. Accessed May 8, 2022.

12. Standring S, Borley NR, et al., eds. *Gray's Anatomy: The Anatomical Basis of Clinical Practice* (40th ed.). London: Churchill Livingstone; 2008:462-464. In: Thyroid. Wikipedia. https://en.wikipedia.org/wiki/Thyroid. Accessed May 8, 2022.

13. Ort V, Bogart BI. *Elsevier's Integrated Anatomy And Embryology*. Philadelphia: Elsevier/Saunders; 2007: 342 In: Thyroid. Wikipedia. https://en.wikipedia.org/wiki/Thyroid. Accessed May 8, 2022.

14. Thyroid. Wikipedia. https://en.wikipedia.org/wiki/Thyroid. Accessed May 8, 2022.

15. Hall JE, Guyton AC. *Guyton and Hall: Textbook of Medical Physiology* (12th ed.). Philadelphia: Saunders/Elsevier; 2011:909. In: Thyroid. Wikipedia. https://en.wikipedia.org/wiki/Thyroid. Accessed May 8, 2022.

16. Sargis RM. How your thyroid works. Endocrineweb.com. In: Thyroid. Wikipedia. https://en.wikipedia.org/wiki/Thyroid. Accessed May 8, 2022.

17. Nussey S, Whitehead S. The thyroid gland. *Endocrinology: An Integrated Approach*. BIOS Scientific Publishers; 2001 In: Thyroid. Wikipedia. https://en.wikipedia.org/wiki/Thyroid. Accessed May 8, 2022.

18. Kocher ET. Concerning pathological manifestations in low-grade thyroid diseases, Nobel Lecture, December 11, 1909:330-383. https://www.nobelprize.org/uploads/2018/06/kocher-lecture.pdf. Accessed May 8, 2022.

19. Voisin A. *Soil, Grass and Cancer.* London: Crosby Lockwood & Sons Ltd.; 1959.

20. Lokhorst G. Descartes and the pineal gland. In: E. N. Zalta, ed. The Stanford Encyclopedia of Philosophy. Winter 2018 Edition. https://plato.stanford.edu/archives/win2018/entries/pineal-gland/. Updated September 18, 2013. Accessed May 8, 2022.

21. Kumar R, Kumar A, Sardhara J. Pineal gland—A spiritual third eye: An odyssey of antiquity to modern chronomedicine. *Indian J Neurosurg*. 2018;7:1-4. DOI 10.1055/s-0038-1649524.

22. Pineal. Online Etymology Dictionary, Douglas Harper. 2018. Retrieved 27 October 2018 In: Pineal Gland. Wikipedia. https://en.wikipedia.org/wiki/Pineal_gland. Accessed May 8, 2022.

23. Ilahi S, Beriwal N, Ilahi TB. Physiology. Pineal Gland. Updated Apr 29, 2021. In: StatPearls. Treasure Island (FL): StatPearls Publishing; 2022. https://www.ncbi.nlm.nih.gov/books/NBK525955/. Accessed May 8, 2022.

24. Aulinas A. Physiology of the pineal gland and melatonin. Updated Dec 10, 2019. In: Feingold KR, Anawalt B, Boyce A, et al., eds. Endotext. South Dartmouth (MA): MDText.com, Inc.; 2000. https://www.ncbi.nlm.nih.gov/books/NBK550972/. Accessed May 8, 2022.

25. Cagnacci A, Elliott JA, Yen SS. Melatonin: A major regulator of the circadian rhythm of core temperature in humans. *J Clin Endocrinol Metab.*1992;75(2):447-452.

26. Standring S, Gray H, eds. *Gray's Anatomy: The Anatomical Basis of Clinical Practice* (41st ed.). Philadelphia. 2016: 983–6. In: Thymus. Wikipedia. https://en.wikipedia.org/wiki/Thymus. Accessed May 8, 2022.

27. Kumar V, Abbas AK, Fausto N, Aster JC. Diseases of white blood cells, lymph nodes, spleen, and thymus. In: *Robbins and Cotran Pathologic Basis of Disease* (9th (online) ed.); 2014. In: Thymus. Wikipedia. https://en.wikipedia.org/wiki/Thymus. Accessed May 8, 2022.

28. Young B, O'Dowd G, Woodford P. *Wheater's Functional Histology: A Text and Colour Atlas* (6th ed.). Philadelphia: Elsevier; 2013:204-206. In: Thymus. Wikipedia. https://en.wikipedia.org/wiki/Thymus. Accessed May 8, 2022.

29. Coller FA, Huggins CB. Effect of hyperthyroidism upon diabetes mellitus: Striking improvement in diabetes mellitus from thyroidectomy. *Annals of Surgery.* 1927: 86(6):877-884.

30. Pancreas. Wikipedia. https://en.wikipedia.org/wiki/Pancreas. Accessed May 8, 2022.

31. Insulin. Wikipedia. https://en.wikipedia.org/wiki/Insulin. Accessed May 8, 2022.

32. Koplik H. Sporadic cretinism and its distinction from forms of idiocy and other diseases. *New York Medical Journal.* Sept 4, 1897.

33. Swain MG. Fatigue in liver disease: Pathophysiology and clinical management. *Can J Gastroenterol.* 2006;20(3):181-188. doi:10.1155/2006/624832.

34. Kidney. Wikipedia. https://en.wikipedia.org/wiki/Kidney. Accessed May 8, 2022.

35. Murray GR. *Diseases of the Thyroid Gland. Part I. Myxoedema and Cretinism.* London: H K Lewis; 1900:34-35

Chapter 9

Medicines—Past and Present

i. Seaweed

The first written record of the use of seaweed for goiter is about 2,000 years ago. Between 200 BC and AD 250, a Chinese book on agriculture and medicinal plants, *The Herbal Classic of the Divine Farmer* (*Chinese: Shennong Ben Cao Jing*), was written. The text was based on a compilation of oral traditions and was a treatise on Chinese herbs and medicine. The original text is said to have been composed of three volumes, containing 365 entries on medicaments and their description.[1] In this book, there is mention of the seaweed *Sargassum* as an efficacious remedy against goiter.[2] It is interesting to note that in one of the earliest known records of thyroid disease, we also find the *medicine*—seaweed. About 1600 years ago, between AD 317 and AD 419, the famous Chinese medical writer Ge-Khun described a mode of treatment for goiter containing seaweeds *Sargassum* and *Laminaria japonica* Aresch.[5] About 900 years ago, between AD 1100 and 1200, there was reference to the use of the seaweed *Laminaria religiosa* Aresch.

Seaweed was also used by people in South America on the Pacific Ocean coast as a medicine for goiter. The Greeks, with a long seacoast, had the same experience, and so did probably all other ancient people who lived on the shores of the sea.[3] Even today, people in Japan, China and Korea consume large amounts of seaweed. They consume seaweed in stews, soups, salads, and in dried form.

What is in seaweed that acts as a medicine for goiter?

ii. Iodine

Seaweed has iodine.

In 1811, the fact that seaweed has iodine was discovered accidently. A chemist and businessman in Paris, Bernard Courtois, was making gunpowder for Napoleon's army. During the Napoleon wars from 1803 to 1815, Napoleon led the French Empire and its allies against other European powers. The many wars created a shortage of wood ashes, the traditional raw material for gunpowder. Wood ashes were used to make potassium nitrate, which was then used to make gunpowder. Because of the shortage of wood ashes, manufacturers of gunpowder switched from wood ashes to seaweed, which was abundantly available on the coasts of France, in Normandy and Brittany.

Like other manufacturers, Bernard Courtois too started making gunpowder from seaweed. One day in 1811, Courtois noticed that there was corrosion of the copper vessels used in the making of gunpowder. He looked for the cause. There was an unusual purple vapor during this corrosion process. The purple vapor later condensed into crystals on coming into contact with cold objects.[4] These new violet-colored crystals were a new element called *iodine*, named after the Greek word for "violet-colored". Thus, iodine was discovered in the process of making gunpowder.

Now, someone had to connect this newly discovered element, iodine, with goiter disease. That someone was Jean-Francois Coindet. Coindet was born in 1774 in Geneva, Switzerland, but his family was originally from a goiter-prone area, Hautie-Savoie, in France. He studied medicine in Edinburgh, Scotland (those days Edinburgh was the pinnacle of the world's medical field), and practiced as a doctor in Geneva, Switzerland.[5] Coindet, through his education, knew that Arnold of Villanova, a physician of 13th century, introduced burned sponge as a treatment for goiter. On July 25th, 1820, Conindet, in his research paper to the Helvetian Society of Natural Sciences assembled at Geneva, made the following observations:

"What is that particular substance in burnt sponge which acts so specifically in goiter? It appeared to me probably that it was iodine. The opinion was confirmed, on my learning that Mr. Fyfe (a Scottish surgeon and chemist), of Edinburgh, had discussed iodine in sponge toward the close of 1819. By this time, I had already witnessed for six months its surprising effects in this goiter malady."[5]

With this seminal research paper, the idea was born that "iodine is a medicine for thyroid disease". Until then, seaweed was the medicine.

Coindet prescribed iodine in the form of potassium iodate to his goiter patients. His recommendation was for mixing 48 grains (3.11 grams) of iodine to one ounce (28.3 ml) of spirits of wine. He instructed his goitrous patients to begin by taking 10 drops three times a day (totaling 1.5 ml per day). This put the initial daily dose at 165 mg iodine, and he recommended gradually doubling this quantity.[5] The recommended duration was for 8–10 weeks. The results of the treatment were spectacular. Shrinking of goiters occurred after 8 days and disappearance or significant improvement of goiters occurred later in many cases.[5] However, in a few patients, the iodine caused severe side effects. These patients suffered from hyperthyroidism symptoms.

Thus, the newly discovered medicine gave birth to another disease, hyperthyroidism. The fear of hyperthyroidism restricted the usage of iodine to short periods of time. After stopping the usage of iodine, goiter appeared again. Because of these side effects, iodine was not commonly used as medicine for another 100 years.

1851

This is a very important year in the history of thyroid disease. In this year, *iodine deficiency* became *the cause* of thyroid disease. Until then, iodine was considered only as a *medicine*.

Chatin, a French chemist, was the first to publish (in 1851) the hypothesis that a *deficiency* of iodine was the actual *cause* of goiter.[5] Chatin, the director of the School of Pharmacy in Paris, had measured iodine in a large number of foodstuffs and water supplies throughout

Western Europe and concluded: "Too low a concentration of iodine in the drinking waters of certain areas appears to be the principal cause of goiter."

After Chatin, other researchers also measured iodine content in drinking water in endemic goiter areas and found these waters to be deficient in iodine. However, there were few other researchers who were not able to confirm the findings that drinking water in endemic goiter areas was deficient in iodine.

1896

Something important happened in the year 1896. Eugene Baumann, a German chemist, found high levels of iodine in the thyroid gland. Eugene Baumann boiled thyroid glands of 1,000 sheep in dilute sulfuric acid and then collected the precipitate that was deposited. While examining the precipitate, he found high levels of iodine in it.[6] This discovery revived the interest in iodine as a medicine for goiter.

1917

The first large-scale experiment was conducted for using iodine as a *preventive medicine* for goiter. This was led by Marine and Kimball in Akron, Ohio, USA.[7] This and similar experiments in Switzerland were the beginning of the use of iodine as *preventive medicine.* Until then, iodine was only used as *medicine when one already had the disease.*

About 5,000 girls, between 11 and 18 years of age took part in the experiment. One group of about 2,200 girls were given a daily dose of 200 mg of sodium iodide in water for 10 days in spring and for 10 days in autumn. That is, in total, 4 grams of iodine was given to each girl over the course of the year. In this group, out of 900 girls with normal thyroid prior to treatment, only 2 (i.e. 0.2%) developed goiter. In the 1,300 girls who had goiter before the start of the experiment, the goiter diminished in size in 60% of the girls.

Another group of 2,300 girls served as controls. These girls were not given any iodine. In this group, out of 1,250 girls with normal thyroid before the experiment, 350 (i.e., 28%) developed goiter. In this group, out of 1,050 girls who had goiter before the start of the experiment, only 14% showed a decrease in the size of the thyroid gland.

Hyperthyroidism was rare in this experiment despite the high level of iodine used. Only 11 cases of hyperthyroidism were reported.

1924

After these successful experiments, iodine was introduced in the community. Iodized salt was introduced on a community scale in four counties in Michigan, in the United States. Table salt containing 1 part iodine in 5,000 parts of salt in the form of potassium iodide was introduced. In the four counties in Michigan, the average goiter rate among the 65,000 school children examined was 39%. Five years later, by 1929, the goiter rate had fallen to 9%. That is, adding iodine to salt as a preventive medicine led to 30 percentage point drop in goiter. No toxic symptoms were observed. Finally, 100 years after the discovery of iodine, iodine started working as a preventive medicine.

1922 – Switzerland

Switzerland was perhaps the first country in the world to add iodine to salt as a *preventive* medicine against goiter and cretinism. In 1922, iodine was added at a dosage of 3.75 mg per kilogram of salt. In 1962, the dosage was doubled to 7.5 mg per kilogram of salt. In 1980, the dosage was again doubled to 15 mg per kilogram of salt. Switzerland arrived at this final dosage through trial and error. The initial dosage was not sufficient to completely address the goiter problem. This was the reason the iodine dosage was increased twice in Switzerland. This preventive measure had enabled Switzerland to prevent goiter and cretinism to a great extent among the Swiss population. Only a small percentage of goiter cases were reported after the 1980 dosage increase. Switzerland is classic example to show that iodine worked as a medicine against goiter and cretinism.

iii. But is Iodine Deficiency the Cause of Goiter and Thyroid Disease?

No. Iodine deficiency is not the cause of thyroid disease.

As we have seen in the previous chapters, it is excess of limestone that is the cause of thyroid disease. Iodine was only acting as a *medicine*.

In addition to iodine, colloid substance in the thyroid gland contains phosphorous, sulphur, arsenic, bromine, and various miscellaneous substances such as leucomains, choline, lipoids, albumosis, xanthin, hypoxanthin, sodium chloride, calcium oxalate, lactic acid, and other substances.[49] But when only iodine is given as a medicine, it creates an imbalance between the level of iodine and the level of all these other substances within the thyroid gland. Such imbalance may result in deranged function of the thyroid gland.

1989

Thyroid disease in Europe persisted despite the addition of iodine to salt in most countries. The following is the summary of an article published in World Health Organization bulletin in 1989. The research for this article was commissioned by the European Thyroid Association and the International Council for Control of Iodine Deficiency Disorders.

"Recent data on iodine excretion in the urine of adults, adolescents, and newborns and iodine content of breastmilk indicate high prevalence of iodine deficiency in many European countries. These cases may manifest themselves as subclinical hypothyroidism."[8]

We can see that almost 50 years after introducing iodine in most European countries, thyroid disease was still highly prevalent in 1989. This shows that iodine may have acted as a medicine for the severe forms of disease—goiter and cretinism. But iodine as a medicine failed to address the subtle and subclinical symptoms of thyroid disease. This leftover subtle thyroid disease is what we now call hypothyroidism. This also shows that iodine may act as a *medicine*, but iodine deficiency is not *the cause* of thyroid disease.

Iodine in the United States

In the United States, iodine has been added to salt for the last 100 years. Yet, medication for hypothyroidism is still among the top three prescriptions. This shows that iodine deficiency is not the cause of thyroid disease. In fact, iodine intake in the United States is excessively high relative to other countries. There is high iodine content in milk in the United States, which is higher than the iodine content of milk in other countries. The United States has a high consumption of fast food and the iodine content in fast food is usually quite high. These facts make it clear that iodine deficiency is not the cause of thyroid disease.

Iodine in Japan

Japan has a long history of consuming high levels of iodine in the form of seaweed. Since ancient times, Japanese have been consuming seaweeds. Yet, Japan is not completely free from thyroid disease, especially in areas with high consumption of seaweed. If iodine deficiency were the cause of thyroid disease, we should not have thyroid disease in these high seaweed consumption areas of Japan. This again implies that iodine deficiency is not the cause of thyroid disease. Iodine only acts as a *medicine.*

Can Iodine Be Harmful?

Yes. Iodine can be harmful.

Anthrax is a fatal disease caused by *Bacillus anthracis,* a bacterium. The disease is usually found in cattle, horses, and sheep. The symptoms of the disease are digestive troubles, intestinal hemorrhage, and the presence of blood or blood cells in urine. Several days after infection, the animals die as a result of suffocation from lack of oxygen. The disease affects human beings who come in contact with the skin or meat of an animal suffering from anthrax. In human beings, the disease begins with a cutaneous lesion (malignant pustule) on the uncovered parts of the body (face, neck, arm, leg) followed by gastrointestinal symptoms (vomiting and diarrhea). In general, human beings are quite resistant to anthrax disease. However, death can occur, usually preceded by convulsions of tetanic (sustained muscle contraction) or epileptic (disruption of nerve cell activity, resulting in seizures) nature.[9]

Anthrax disease has been known since antiquity. It is known to have caused considerable losses among cattle in the 19th century. Various causes were given for anthrax disease—bad pastures, bad irrigation water, weather factors, bad fodder, and dirty stables. However, Casimir Davaine (1812–1882), a little-known French physician, was instrumental in our understanding that anthrax is caused by a *microbe,* a bacterium. And the treatment recommended by Casimir Davaine for such a deadly anthrax disease? Iodine.

Davaine, in one of his last papers to the Academy of Medicine in 1880, considered treatment of human anthrax by iodine. Iodine can be useful in killing anthrax in humans. So, iodine as a medicine is fine when we are attacked by this bacterium. But what about rest of the time when we are not likely to be attacked by such bacterium? Would taking iodine in small doses in the form of iodized salt every day with every meal be harmful?

We know today that we have trillions of beneficial bacteria, virus, and fungi in the intestines and other areas of the human body. It is called human microbiome. What impact does iodine have on the trillions of beneficial bacteria, virus, and fungi? Just like many things in medicine, iodine is both useful and harmful. The dose determines the usefulness or harmfulness. The iodine taken via salt all over the world is in very minute quantities. Further research is needed to know if iodine even in such minute quantities over the life of an individual can be harmful.

Antonio Grossich (1849–1926), a Croatia surgeon, was among the first to use sterilization of the operative field. In 1908, he introduced tincture of iodine to rapidly sterilize the human skin in the surgical field.[10] So, once again we see that iodine was used as a disinfectant. Iodine kills bad bacteria. But when taken regularly, does iodine kill the good bacteria too in the intestines?

In chemistry, iodine belongs to a group of chemicals called halogens. Chlorine, fluorine, bromine, and iodine are halogens, and all are related chemically. One common function of halogens is that they are used for disinfection. There is a relationship between infection and thyroid disease. Iodine may be working in thyroid disease because of its property as a disinfectant. In addition, supplemental iodine may be providing iodine to thyroid gland, which has one of the highest reserves of iodine and is essential for the production of thyroid hormones.

Iodine Excess and Thyroid Autoimmunity

Excess iodine in food, water, and drugs results in disturbances of thyroid function and goiter.[11,12] We may note that iodine at appropriate levels acts as a medicine and at excess levels causes goiter. Clinical data as well as animal experiences have shown a sharp rise in the incidence of autoimmune thyroiditis when iodine consumption was increased.[12,13,14] Administration of iodine or iodine-containing drugs increases the incidence of thyroid autoantibodies in humans without illness as well as in populations with endemic goiter.[15,16,17]

The thyroid gland makes a protein called thyroglobulin. It is used to produce thyroid hormones. When someone consumes excess iodine, weapons/antibodies may be generated that destroy thyroglobulin. This is how intake of excess iodine disrupts the functioning of the thyroid gland.

Similarly, the thyroid gland has an enzyme called thyroid peroxide. Thyroid peroxide also plays an important role in the production of thyroid hormones. When someone consumes excess iodine, antibodies may be generated by the body that destroy this enzyme.

We thus see that consumption of excess iodine disrupts the functioning of the thyroid gland by destroying the proteins and enzymes in the gland.

The antibodies in our blood are measured using a diagnostic test called radioimmune assay. As we have seen previously, there is a fine interplay of many hormones in the body of a woman as a result of the hormonal changes at puberty, pregnancy, breast-feeding, and menopause. When the fine interplay of hormones is disrupted by addition of synthetic/man-made iodine in the diet, women are more likely to suffer from autoimmune symptoms.

In Tasmania, Australia, about three months after the addition of iodate to bread, there was a startling increase in the incidence of thyrotoxicosis in middle-aged and elderly people.[18] The form of iodine added to bread was the likely culprit. And more so because, even before addition of iodine to bread, Australians in general were consuming high levels of iodine in the form of dairy products and the use of iodine-based disinfectants in the milk industry.

In studies in Sarawak, Malaysia, a striking increase in the incidence of thyrotoxicosis was found after iodine was introduced.[19]

The Form of Iodine Matters

The diet in Japan customarily includes large quantities of foods rich in iodine, and the average daily intake of iodine is several milligrams. However, the quantity and the frequency of ingestion of these foods vary greatly. Some people ingest 20 milligrams (mg) of iodine per day, and others only 100 micrograms (μg). That is, some people consume 200 times more than others (20 milligrams vs. 100 micrograms). Some people ingest large quantities everyday while others only once every several months. The source of dietary iodine is seaweeds, especially tangle. Yet, hyperthyroidism is rare among the Japanese. On the other hand, in Europe, only a minute amount of iodine is added to salt, and yet Europe has large number of hyperthyroidism and thyrotoxicosis cases. Perhaps the form of iodine is the cause of the distinct results between Japan and Europe. In Japan, naturally occurring iodine in seaweed is consumed, whereas in Europe, artificially made potassium iodide is used.

In Japan, a patient was given Aminodarone, an iodine-rich drug to treat irregular heartbeat. When the patient was withdrawn from the drug, he developed severe hyperthyroidism symptoms.[20] There are a large number of such cases where people suffer from hyperthyroidism symptoms when they are taken off iodine-rich medication. That is not to say that there is no harm from seaweeds. There have been reports of iodine-induced hypothyroidism and hyperthyroidism in kelp-consuming populations of Japan.

The seaweeds that Bernard Courtois used in discovering iodine (and the ash obtained on burning them) contains chlorides, bromides, iodides, carbonates, and sulfates of sodium, potassium, magnesium, and calcium. In his day, however, seaweeds were valued merely for their sodium and potassium compounds, which were recovered by burning the dried algae.[21] As we can see, seaweed and burned sponge did not contain merely iodine; they contained a large number of other minerals too. When people were eating seaweed as a medicine for goiter, they were getting these are minerals too along with iodine. For example, they were also getting bromine when they ate seaweed. But not much research was done to find out whether bromine was deficient in the drinking waters in the goiter endemic regions. Researchers just looked for iodine in endemic regions; they did not look for bromine. It is quite probable that bromine was also deficient in all the goiter-producing waters. This again shows that it is not iodine *deficiency* which is *the cause* of goiter and thyroid disease. As we have seen previously, it is the *excess* limestone in water which is the cause of thyroid disease.

Iodine in the Human Body

Iodine is present in many other organs and tissues of the body—in nervous system, lungs, liver, kidneys, adrenals, bile, muscles, spleen, lymph glands, hair, pituitary, thymus, and nuclei of all cells.[22] In no other tissue or organ, however, does it exist in such quantities as in the thyroid gland. In the other organs just mentioned, it never forms more than 0.001%, whereas in the thyroid, the minimum amount necessary for health is 0.01%, and a maximum quantity of 1.16% has been recorded, i.e., iodine in the thyroid gland is ten to hundred times more than in other organs.[21]

Under normal conditions the diet always contains sufficient iodine for the upkeep of this minimal amount.[21] Iodine exits in the thyroid in organic combination with amino acid groups. It is present in a proportion of 0.3%–0.9% per gram of the dried gland. The adult gland contains 2–9 mg of iodine. As noted earlier, the iodine content varies with age, diet, season, and sex. Female animals have relatively more iodine per unit of body weight than do males.

Therefore, while iodine is an important constituent of thyroid gland and acts as medicine or preventive medicine, it is required in a very minute quantity. The form of iodine taken is also important. The synthetic/man-made iodine that we take through iodized salt and iodine supplements and in excess over time may lead to autoimmune thyroid symptoms, hyperthyroidism, and thyroid-toxicity.

iv. Animal Thyroid

Our ancestors were good observers. They tried to treat the neck swelling in humans with a medicine made from the necks of animals. They used the thyroid gland of animals to cure thyroid disease in man.

Again, it is from China that we have the first recorded use of animal thyroid for the treatment of goiter disease. Between AD 420 and 501, the use of deer thyroid in the treatment of goiter is mentioned in the Chinese book *Shen-Fan*. The Chinese treated "cretinism" with sheep's thyroid in the sixth century.[23] Thus, for both goiter and cretinism, animal thyroid was used as a medicine in China at least 1,500 years ago. The Chinese prepared this medicine by taking the thyroid glands of 100 sheep, washing them, drying them, and making pills out of them.[24] There are references to the use of animal thyroid in China for the next thousand years (i.e., from AD 500 to AD 1500). In the Ming Dynasty (AD 1552 to 1578), the Chinese physician Li Shi-Chen mentioned preparations of pig and deer thyroid in the treatment of thyroid diseases.

In modern times, animal thyroid gland (in the form of desiccated/dried thyroid gland) has been used since the late 1800s.[25] In the 1890s, William Ord undertook some of the earliest studies of the effects of treating hypothyroidism (myxedema) with animal thyroid extract.[26] Treatment with animal thyroid extract led to rapid weight loss, rise in temperature, increase in urinary volume, and increase in nitrogen excretion.[27] All these are symptoms of hyperthyroidism. So, again the medicine for one disease, hypothyroidism, created a new disease, hyperthyroidism.

In 1891, in Britain, George Murray, treated a case of hypothyroidism (myxoedema) with an extract of sheep's thyroid given through an injection. He treated four such patients and published his research in

1892. After Murray's research, there were reports from others of success with thyroid extract taken orally. However, overdose was common, patients suffered from fast-beating heart, rise in pulse, and rise in body temperature, which are all symptoms of hyperthyroidism. Therefore, as with iodine, getting the right dose of animal thyroid was difficult.

Desiccated/dried thyroid sold today is normally made from the thyroids of pigs, sheep, or cows.[28] In 2017, it was the 130th most prescribed medication in the United States, with more than 5 million prescriptions.[29,30] Usage has decreased since the 1960s, with increasing use of synthetic thyroid hormone.[31]

v. Synthetic Thyroid Hormone

Animal thyroid as a medicine had a few drawbacks such as inconsistent dosage and inconsistent quality. To address these drawbacks, pharmaceutical companies started making thyroid hormone in their factories. This factory-made thyroid, i.e., synthetic thyroid hormone, is what most thyroid patients today take as medicine for hypothyroidism. While it is easier to make synthetic thyroid hormone in a factory, the reason more people are put on thyroid medication today than in earlier times is the development of a new diagnostic test. This diagnostic test measures the thyroid stimulating hormone (TSH). The TSH diagnostic test became widely available in 1970s.

The TSH, although it has the word "thyroid" in the name, is actually released by the pituitary gland. As the name says, the Thyroid Stimulating Hormone *stimulates* the thyroid gland to produce thyroid hormones. In hypothyroidism, there is excess of thyroid stimulating hormone (TSH) in the blood.

The new TSH diagnostic test in the 1970s showed that people who were taking animal thyroid extracts were taking it in excess. To address this problem, synthetic thyroid hormone was produced in factories to ensure consistent dosage.

Thyroid Hormones Produced by Thyroid Gland—T_4, T_3, and Calcitonin

Before we discuss synthetic thyroid hormone, let us briefly discuss the thyroid hormones secreted naturally by the thyroid gland.

Of the three hormones produced by thyroid gland, the major hormone is T_4, which is also called thyroxine. In 1915, it was first isolated by the American chemist Edward Kendall.[32] In 1926, its chemical structure was determined by Harington.[33] In 1927, it was first synthesized (made artificially) by Harington and Barger.[34]

The other major hormone produced by the thyroid gland is triiodothyronine (T_3). In 1952–53, T_3 was identified, isolated, and synthesized by Gross and Pitt-Rivers.[35,36] T_3 is the true hormone.[37] It is 3–4 times more potent than T_4.

In humans, a normal thyroid gland produces ~85 mcg of T_4 and 6.5 mcg of T_3 daily.[38,39] Thus, the ratio of T_4:T_3 that is directly secreted from the thyroid gland is around 13:1. The remaining daily T_3 production, about 26.5 mcg, is derived from the conversion of T_4. Microgram or mcg is a unit of mass equal to one-millionth of a gram. Are all the symptoms of hypothyroidism caused because of changes at the level of one-millionth of a gram in thyroid hormone secretion?

T_4 is converted to the active T_3 within cells by selenium-containing enzymes, and thus dietary selenium is essential for T_3 production. The major portion of T_3 is produced in peripheral organs[40] (e.g., liver, adipose tissue, glia, and skeletal muscle) from circulating T_4. This process is controlled by numerous hormones and nerval signals, including TSH, vasopressin, and catecholamines. The circulating T_3 is formed, for example, in the liver and the pituitary by removal of the iodine atom from the carbon atom number five of the outer ring of T_4. But what happens when we artificially supply excess iodine in the form of iodized salt? Does the excess iodine disrupt the process of conversion from T_4 to T_3?

Levothyroxine

Levothyroxine is the factory-made version of T_4. In 1949, Glaxo pharmaceutical company made the commercially available levothyroxine. It is this form of thyroid hormone that is prescribed today all over the world for hypothyroidism. Even though thyroxine became commercially available in 1949, tablets of desiccated/dried animal thyroid extract remained the principal source of treatment for many years.[41]

The factory-made thyroid hormone, levothyroxine, has only thyroxine (T_4). Animal thyroid hormones derived from pig thyroid glands contain 20% T_3 and traces of T_2, T_1, and calcitonin.

In summary, a new diagnostic test, TSH, brought in large number of new thyroid patients and these new patients were given the factory-made thyroid hormone. The world has been, and is still, on this path for the last 50 years. The TSH test has been so successful in bringing in new patients that sales of levothyroxine, the artificially made thyroid hormone, is among the top three prescription drugs in the United States. If there was no TSH test, perhaps not many patients would have been put on this synthetic drug.

Drug Approval Process Was Skipped for Levothyroxine

Today, if any new medicine/drug must be launched in the United States, it usually goes through a lengthy approval process. The new drug approval process takes about 12 years from idea to commercial launch. Before a new drug is launched, it is first tested in animals, then tested for safety among a small number of human volunteers, and then in phases tested for efficacy among a larger set of patients.

Levothyroxine did not go through this lengthy process. It was introduced as a replacement for animal thyroid in 1950s. And then it continued to be used among patients. Per the US Food and Drug Administration definition, levothyroxine sodium was an *unapproved marketed drug* before the year 2000.[42] After the year 2000, per US FDA guidelines, levothyroxine manufacturers had to test only for whether patients were getting the dose as advertised on the label.

As in the case of iodine, levothyroxine also works as a medicine for a few symptoms of low thyroid disease. There are certain positive improvements like less brain fog, fewer infections, and weight loss. But ask any person who is taking levothyroxine how they feel. You would not get a positive response. The side effects of levothyroxine can be severe. The skin becomes moist and soft and losses its shine, the hair becomes brittle and falls out, the heart rate increases. It is not possible to withdraw from the thyroid medication. Withdrawal could lead to hyperthyroidism symptoms, rapid heartbeat, rapid nervous function, extreme agitation, significant weight loss, muscle loss, and so on. Hyperthyroidism can be fatal in extreme cases. It is better to live with hypothyroidism than suffer from hyperthyroidism.

The proper dosage for iodine was arrived at after about 100 years of trial and error. I believe that a similar process of trial and error is underway for levothyroxine.

vi. Surgery

When a surgeon removes the thyroid gland in goiter disease, he is just removing a visible symptom. He is not addressing the underlying disease. We have seen in previous chapters that thyroid disease affects the whole body, not just the gland. Surgery does not address the acid-base imbalance or disease in the other glands of the body.

In thyroid disease, the other glands of the body are also involved, e.g., the pituitary gland, adrenal glands. But the disease in these other glands is not as easily visible as enlargement of the thyroid gland. Hence, surgery has historically been restricted to the thyroid gland. We do not hear much about surgery for pituitary gland or pineal gland.

The earliest reference of surgical treatment of goiter was a thousand years ago, around the year AD 952. This reference to thyroid surgery is mentioned in *Kitāb al-Taṣrīf* ("The Arrangement of Medical Knowledge for One Who is Not Able to Compile a Book for Himself"), a 30-volume Arabic encyclopedia on medicine and surgery, written by Abu al-Qasim al-Zahrawi (Abulcasis).[43] His experience with thyroid surgery was recorded in the book as *removal of a large goiter under sedation with opium.*[44]

For the next 800 years, thyroid surgery was done for goiter, but the death rate after these surgeries was quite high. Death rates were high because surgery was primitive in earlier times, and complications often arose due to blood loss during surgery and infections after surgery. Such complications were common in all types of surgeries, not just thyroid surgery. But the death rate in thyroid surgery was especially high.

In the context of thyroid surgery, William Stewart Halsted (1852–1922), a US surgeon, in his "The operative history of goiter," scrutinized procedures done before 1850 and noted them to be associated with 40% mortality.[44] The French Academy of Medicine banned thyroid surgery in 1850 because of the high mortality associated with them.[44] Many prominent surgeons of the day, such as Robert Liston (British surgeon, 1794–1847) and Samuel Gross (American surgeon, 1805–1884), did not recommend surgery for goiter. The predominant view on thyroid surgery is best summarized by the American surgeon Samuel Gross: "No honest and sensible surgeon would ever engage in it."[44]

With time, there were advances in surgery. Better surgical techniques led to less loss of blood during the surgery; excessive loss of blood during thyroid surgery was one of the key reasons for the high mortality rates. Sterilization of surgical instruments led to fewer infections.

Many stalwarts of surgery contributed to bringing down the mortality associated with thyroid surgery. However, two surgeons need special mention—Theodor Billroth and Theodor Kocher. It is no surprise that both these surgeons did their work in Switzerland, the epicenter of thyroid disease research in 1800s, and also the epicenter of severe thyroid disease.

Theodor Billroth (1829–1894) was a giant of 19th century surgery. He worked in Zurich, Switzerland, and noted endemic goiter in his surroundings. He instituted surgery for goiter to address various symptoms associated with goiter disease. He got disheartened when 40% of his patients died (8 died out of 20 patients), and so he suspended surgery as a treatment for goiter.[45] Six years later, he moved to Vienna, Austria, another endemic goiter region. With better management of anesthesia, blood loss, and infection, Billroth tried again. The mortality rate dropped to less than 10%. He was on a path to become the most-practiced thyroid surgeon worldwide.[45]

Theodor Kocher (1841–1917) was a student of Billroth. With obsessive diligence and focus, Kocher further reduced blood loss and infections during thyroid surgery to a minimal. As a result, he was able to bring down thyroid surgery mortality rate to 0.2% by 1898. In his lifetime, Kocher performed over 5,000 surgeries, with mortality rate of 0.5%. Under his tenure, Berne, Switzerland, became the global capital of thyroid surgery. Kocher was awarded the Nobel Prize in 1909 for his work on thyroid surgery and furthering our understanding of the functioning of the thyroid gland. Yet, the most successful thyroid surgeon of the world was unhappy with his work. His patients did not become better, they often became worse after the surgery.

Kocher noted that after surgery the patients became *physically sluggish* and *mentally slow*. He noted cretinism symptoms post-operation—dry skin, coarse features, slothful demeanor, and mental retardation. Kocher, in describing his 11-year-old patient observed: "She has become peevish and dull and will not work except under compulsion, whereas formerly she was a spirited and joyous creature."[45] Kocher summarized: "In technical terms, we have certainly learned to master the operation for goiter. But removal of the thyroid gland has deprived my patients of what gives them human value. I have doomed people with goiter, otherwise healthy, to a vegetative existence. Many of them I have turned to cretins, saved them for a life not worth living."[45]

Because of these complications, Kocher advised not to remove the thyroid gland completely, but to remove only one side/part of the thyroid gland. One of his famous rules read "A surgeon is a doctor who can operate and also knows when not to."

We have to heed the advice of history's best thyroid surgeon—*not to do the thyroid surgery when it is not required.* As we have seen through most of this book, thyroid disease is a disease of the whole body, and not just the gland. Surgery does not address underlying the disease, the acid–base imbalance.

The only exception may be when there is cancer in the thyroid gland. Further research is required in the field of thyroid cancer. But a brief note may be made on cancer in general.

In 1909, an English surgeon, Stuart-Low, stated that he had never seen cancer in a patient suffering from hypothyroidism (myxedema).[46] This has been my personal observation too. I have researched considerable literature in the process of writing this book, I have hardly come across any references to cancer in goiter, cretinism, or hypothyroid patients. On the other hand, Stuart-Low observed that an increased secretion of thyroxine, T_4 (hyperthyroidism), aided the development of tumors/cancer. It is possible that the overall reduced metabolism brought about by hypothyroidism may be reducing the metabolism of even cancerous cells and thereby causing less cancer. The increased metabolism when excess thyroid hormone (thyroxine) is secreted (e.g., as in hyperthyroidism) quite likely increases the metabolism of even cancerous cells.

If this hypothesis is true, then we should have overall less cancer in lime/chalk districts. We have evidence supporting this phenomenon. In 1868, Haviland reported to the Medical Society of London that it was possible that the soil exerts some influence on the frequency of cancer.[47] Examining the relationship between cancer frequency and the geological map of England and Wales, he concluded that cancer frequency was greater on clay soils prone to seasonal flooding by large rivers. Chalk countries were remarkably free from cancer.

However, data conflicting the above hypothesis on the relationship between goiter and cancer was noted by a few other researchers. According to Berard and Dunet and their work on the thyroid cancer, in goiter-free districts, there were 4–5 malignant/cancer thyroid glands in 1,000 pathological tumors (a tumor is an abnormal mass of tissue that may or may not become cancerous), while in goitrous regions, there were 25–40 malignant/cancer thyroid glands.[48]

As noted earlier, further research is required on the topic of thyroid cancer.

Caution: The purpose of the above discussion is to provide information and analysis. It is not intended to be medical advice. I am not a medical doctor. You should consult your physician for medical advice. Every patient is unique and his or her circumstances are unique. Only your physician will be able to advice the best approach for your specific needs and circumstances.

References

1. Shennong Ben Cao Jing. Wikipedia. https://en.wikipedia.org/wiki/Shennong_Ben_Cao_Jing. Accessed May 8, 2022.
2. Langer P. History of Goiter. In: *Endemic Goiter.* Monograph Series No. 44. Geneva: World Health Organization; 1960:9.
3. Matovinovic J, Ramalingaswami V. Therapy and prophylaxis of endemic goiter. In: *Endemic Goiter.* Monograph Series No. 44. Geneva: World Health Organization; 1960:385.
4. Swain PA. Bernard Courtois (1777-1838), famed for discovering Iodine (1811) and his life in Paris from 1798. *Bull Hist Chem.* 2005;30(2):103-111. http://acshist.scs.illinois.edu/awards/OPA%20Papers/2007-Swain.pdf. Accessed on May 8, 2022.
5. Orgiazzi J, Spaulding SW. Milestones in European thyroidology: Jean-Francois Coindet (1774-1834). https://www.eurothyroid.com/about/met/coindet.html. Accessed on May 8, 2022.
6. Niazi AK, Kalra S, Irfan A, Islam A. Thyroidology over ages. *Indian J Endocrinol Metab.* 2011; 15(6):121-126.
7. Matovinovic J, Ramalingaswami V. Therapy and prophylaxis of endemic goiter. In: *Endemic Goiter.* Monograph Series No. 44. Geneva: World Health Organization; 1960:387.
8. Delange F, Burgi H. Iodine deficiency disorders in Europe. *Bull World Health Org.* 1989;67(3): 317-325.

9. Theodorides J. Casimir Davaine (1812-1882): The precursor of Pastuer. A Lecture given on May 10, 1965, at the Wellcome Historical Medical Library, London. doi: 10.1017/s0025727300010942.

10. Iodine. Wikipedia. https://en.wikipedia.org/wiki/Iodine. Accessed May 8, 2022.

11. Pennington JAT. A view of iodine toxicity reports. *J Amer Diet Assoc.* 1990:90:1571. In: Matsuura N, Harada S. Iodine Excess and Thyroid Autoimmunity. In: Delange F, Dunn JT, Glinoer D, eds. *Iodine Deficiency in Europe.* NATO ASI Series (Series A: Life Sciences). New York & London: Plenum Press; 1993:93-99.

12. Fradkin JE, Wolff J. Iodide-induced thyrotoxicosis. *Medicine.* 1983:62:1. In: Matsuura N, Harada S. Iodine Excess and Thyroid Autoimmunity. In: Delange F, Dunn JT, Glinoer D, eds. *Iodine Deficiency in Europe.* NATO ASI Series (Series A: Life Sciences). New York & London: Plenum Press; 1993:93-99.

13. Bagchi N, Brown TR, Urdanivia E, Sundick RS. Induction of autoimmune thyroiditis in chickens by dietary iodine. *Science.* 1985:230:325. In: Matsuura N, Harada S. Iodine Excess and Thyroid Autoimmunity. In: Delange F, Dunn JT, Glinoer D, eds. *Iodine Deficiency in Europe.* NATO ASI Series (Series A: Life Sciences). New York & London: Plenum Press; 1993:93-99.

14. Allen EL, Appel MC, Braverman LE. The effect of iodide ingestion on the development of spontaneous lymphocytic thyroiditis in the diabetes-prone BB/W rat. *J Clin Endocrinol Metab.* 1986;118:1977. In: Matsuura N, Harada S. Iodine Excess and Thyroid Autoimmunity. In: Delange F, Dunn JT, Glinoer D, eds. *Iodine Deficiency in Europe.* NATO ASI Series (Series A: Life Sciences). New York & London: Plenum Press; 1993:93-99.

15. Harach HR, Escalante DA, Onativia A, Outes JL, Day S, Williams E. Thyroid carcinoma and thyroiditis in an endemic goiter region before and after iodine prophylaxis. *Acta Endocrinol.* 1985;108:55. In: Matsuura N, Harada S. Iodine Excess and Thyroid

Autoimmunity. In: Delange F, Dunn JT, Glinoer D, eds. *Iodine Deficiency in Europe*. NATO ASI Series (Series A: Life Sciences). New York & London: Plenum Press; 1993:93-99.

16. Ford HC, Johnson LA, Feek CM, Newton JD. Iodine intake and the seasonal incidence of thyrotoxicosis in New Zealand. *Clin Endocrinol.* 1991;34:179. In: Matsuura N, Harada S. Iodine Excess and Thyroid Autoimmunity. In: Delange F, Dunn JT, Glinoer D, eds. *Iodine Deficiency in Europe.* NATO ASI Series (Series A: Life Sciences). New York & London: Plenum Press; 1993:93-99.
17. Monteiro E, Galvao-Teles A, Santos ML, et al. Antithyroid antibodies as an early marker for thyroid disease induced by amiodarone. *Brit Med J.* 1986:292:227. In: Matsuura N, Harada S. Iodine Excess and Thyroid Autoimmunity. In: Delange F, Dunn JT, Glinoer D, eds. *Iodine Deficiency in Europe.* NATO ASI Series (Series A: Life Sciences). New York & London: Plenum Press; 1993:93-99.
18. Connolly RJ, Stewart TC, Vidor G. An increase in thyrotoxicosis in an endemic goiter area following iodisation of bread. *Lancet.* 1970;1:500-503. In: Eastman CJ. The Status of Iodine Nutrition in Australia. Delange F, Dunn JT, Glinoer D, eds. *Iodine Deficiency in Europe.* NATO ASI Series (Series A: Life Sciences). New York & London: Plenum Press; 1993.
19. Eastman CJ. The Status of iodine nutrition in Australia. In: Delange F, Dunn JT, Glinoer D, eds. *Iodine Deficiency in Europe.* NATO ASI Series (Series A: Life Sciences). New York & London: Plenum; 1993:139.
20. Braverman LE. Thyroid Dysfunction induced by excess iodine. In: Delange F, Dunn JT, Glinoer D, eds. *Iodine Deficiency in Europe.* NATO ASI Series (Series A: Life Sciences). New York & London: Plenum; 1993:82-83.
21. Mary EW, *The Discovery of the Elements*, 1934.
22. McCarrison R. *The Thyroid Gland in Health and Disease.* New York: William Wood & Company. 1917:17-18.

23. Hume EH. The contributions of China to the science and art of medicine. *Science* 1924;59:345–50. In: Slater S. The discovery of thyroid replacement therapy, Part 1: In the beginning, *J R Soc Med.* 2011:104: 15–18. DOI 10.1258/jrsm.2010.10k050.

24. Slater S. The discovery of thyroid replacement therapy, Part 1: In the beginning, *J R Soc Med.* 2011;104:15-18. DOI 10.1258/jrsm.2010.10k050.

25. Jameson JL, Groot LJ. *Endocrinology: Adult and Pediatric* (*e-Book*). Elsevier; 2010:1608. In: Desiccated Thyroid. Wikipedia. https://en.wikipedia.org/wiki/Desiccated_thyroid_extract. Accessed May 8, 2022.

26. Slater S. The discovery of thyroid replacement therapy, Part 2: The critical 19th century, *J R Soc Med.* 2011;104: 59-63. DOI 10.1258/jrsm.2010.10k051.

27. Ord WM, White E. Clinical remarks on certain changes observed in the urine in myxoedema after the administration of glycerine extract of thyroid gland. *BMJ.* 1893;ii:217. In: Slater S. The discovery of thyroid replacement therapy, Part 2: The critical 19th century, *J R Soc Med.* 2011: 104: 59–63. DOI 10.1258/jrsm.2010.10k051.

28. Thomas JA, Keenan EJ. *Principles of Endocrine Pharmacology. Springer Science & Business Media.* 2021:78. In: Desiccated Thyroid. Wikipedia. https://en.wikipedia.org/wiki/Desiccated_thyroid_extract. Accessed May 8, 2022.

29. "The top 300 of 2020". ClinCalc. Retrieved 11 April 2020. In: Desiccated Thyroid. Wikipedia. https://en.wikipedia.org/wiki/Desiccated_thyroid_extract. Accessed May 8, 2022. .

30. "Thyroid—Drug usage statistics". ClinCalc. Retrieved 11 April 2020. In: Desiccated Thyroid. Wikipedia. https://en.wikipedia.org/wiki/Desiccated_thyroid_extract. Accessed May 8, 2022.

31. Larry JJ, Leslie GJ. *Endocrinology - E-Book: Adult and Pediatric. Elsevier Health Sciences*; 2010:1608. In: Desiccated Thyroid.

Wikipedia. https://en.wikipedia.org/wiki/Desiccated_thyroid_extract. Accessed May 8, 2022.

32. Kendall EC. The isolation in crystalline form of the compound containing iodin, which occurs in the thyroid: its chemical nature and physiologic activity. *J. Am Med Ass.* 1915;64:2042-2043. In: Slater S. The discovery of thyroid replacement therapy, Part 3: In the beginning, *J R Soc Med.* 2010:104:100–106. DOI 10.1258/jrsm.2010.10k052.

33. Harington CR. Chemistry of thyroxine. II: Constitution and synthesis of desiodo-thyroxine. *Biochem J.* 1926;20:300-313. In: Slater S. The discovery of thyroid replacement therapy, Part 3: In the beginning, *J R Soc Med.* 2010:104:100–106. DOI 10.1258/jrsm.2010.10k052.

34. Harington CR, Barger G. Chemistry of thyroxine. III: Constitution and synthesis of thyroxine. *Biochem J.* 1927;21:169-183. In: Slater S. The discovery of thyroid replacement therapy, Part 3: In the beginning, *J R Soc Med* 2010: 104: 100–106. DOI 10.1258/jrsm.2010.10k052.

35. Gross J, Pitt-Rivers R. The identification of 3:5:3# -Ltriiodothyronine in human plasma. *Lancet.* 1952;i:439-441. In: Slater S. The discovery of thyroid replacement therapy, Part 3: In the beginning, J R Soc Med 2010: 104: 100–106. DOI 10.1258/jrsm.2010.10k052.

36. Gross J, Pitt-Rivers R. 3:5:3# Triiodothyronine. I: Isolation from thyroid gland and synthesis. *Biochem J.* 1953;53:645-652. in Slater S. The discovery of thyroid replacement therapy, Part 3: In the beginning, *J R Soc Med.* 2010: 104: 100–106. DOI 10.1258/jrsm.2010.10k052.

37. Triiodothyronine. Wikipedia. https://en.wikipedia.org/wiki/Triiodothyronine. Accessed May 8, 2022.

38. Gomes-Lima C et. al. Can reverse T3 assay be employed to guide T4 vs. T4/T3 therapy in hypothyroidism? *Front Endocrinol.* 11 December 2019. https://doi.org/10.3389/fendo.2019.00856.

39. Jonklaas J, Bianco AC, Bauer AJ, Burman KD, Cappola AR, Celi FS, et al. Guidelines for the treatment of hypothyroidism (prepared by the American Thyroid Association task force on thyroid hormone replacement). *Thyroid.* (2014) 24;1670-751. doi: 10.1089/thy.2014.0028. In: Gomes-Lima C et. al. Can reverse T3 assay be employed to guide T4 vs. T4/T3 therapy in hypothyroidism? *Front Endocrinol.* 11 December 2019. https://doi.org/10.3389/fendo.2019.00856.

40. Hypothalamic–pituitary–thyroid axis. Wikipedia. https://en.wikipedia.org/wiki/Hypothalamic-pituitary-thyroid_axis. Accessed May 8, 2022.

41. Slater S. The discovery of thyroid replacement therapy, Part 3: In the beginning, *J R Soc Med.* 2010;104:100-106. DOI 10.1258/jrsm.2010.10k052.

42. Malinowski H. Bioavailability/bioequivalence studies in evaluation of new levothyroxine products. FDA. https://www.fda.gov/media/77811/download. Accessed May 8, 2022.

43. Al-Tasrif. Wikipedia. https://en.wikipedia.org/wiki/Al-Tasrif. Accessed May 8, 2022.

44. Sarkar S, Banerjee S, Sarkar R, Sikder B. A Review on the History of 'Thyroid Surgery'. *Indian J Surg.* 2016;78(1):32-36. doi:10.1007/s12262-015-1317-5.

45. Hannan AS. The magnificent seven: a history of modern thyroid surgery. *Intl J Surgery.* 2006;4:3:187-191 DOI: 10.1016/j.ijsu.2006.03.002.

46. Stuart-Low W. *Lancet.* 1909;177(2),1138-1140. In: Voisin A. *Soil, Grass and Cancer.* London: Crosby Lockwood & Son Ltd; 1959.

47. Haviland A. *Brit Med J.* November 26, 1870. In: Voisin A. *Soil, Grass and Cancer.* London: Crosby Lockwood & Son Ltd; 1959.

48. Bram I. *Exophthalmic Goitre and Its Nonsurgical Treatment.* St. Louis: C V Mosby Company; 1920:40.

Chapter 10

The Cure

The cure becomes self-evident when we have found the cause. Limestone-source water is the cause of thyroid disease. The cure for the disease is to change the drinking water source to a non–limestone-source. There can be no cure without change of the drinking water source.

About a thousand years ago, Arnold de Villanova (1235–1312), who practiced as a physician in Spain, France, and Italy, advised those suffering from goiter that they migrate to another region if they were less than 25 years of age.[1] The advice remains the same today. One should change one's location if one is suffering from severe thyroid disease and only limestone water or hard water is available in their present home/location. Alternately, one may get water for drinking and cooking purposes from a nearby non–limestone-water source.

In the goiter-affected villages in the Himalayas in India, people "lost" their goiter on changing their location to a non-goitrous locality. At a French boarding school, students lost their goiters when they were on vacation, i.e., when they changed their source of drinking water. Similarly, tourists to a few French destinations got "holiday goiter" when they were on vacation and lost the goiter shortly after the holidays, i.e., when they went back to their non-goitrous water source.

When one is unable to get non–limestone-source water in their area, the next best alternative is to boil the water before drinking or using for cooking purposes. This results in the lime (calcium carbonate) in water depositing itself on the surface of the utensils. This way, there will be less lime in the water. This works because of lime's (calcium carbonate's) property of retrograde solubility. Just as calcium carbonate dissolves more easily in water in the winter season, boiling water would make calcium carbonate less soluble in water. Hence, warm/boiled water has less lime in it.

Thyroid Gland Can Recover

About 1838, it was noted that the use of waters from certain sources in the Alps mountains (Department Léman in the hamlet of Thuet) produced goiter in 8 or 10 days.[2] In China, immigrant Japanese rapidly became victims; a Japanese noncommissioned officer acquired goiter 4 months after entering the country, and a consular police official contracted a second-degree thyroid enlargement within 9 months of being stationed at Pingchuan.[3] In India, McClelland observed that goiter takes 6 years or more to reach its full size.[4]

Therefore, people coming into a goiter location take a few days, months, or years in developing the disease. A similar time period may be required to "lose" the goiter. Goiters of long-standing could take more time to dissolve. We have seen in villages near Lohaghat (villages # 7 to 15 in Chapter 4) that severe cases of long-standing goiter may not be resolved despite change in location and source of water. In few cases, it was noted that goiter related symptoms subsided only by the third generation after a family moved out of a goitrous location. That is, the second generation of the family still had goiter related symptoms even through the family moved out of a goitrous location.

As in goiter, even in the case of hypothyroidism, the time taken for resolving hypothyroidism symptoms may depend on the time one was exposed to hypothyroidism disease-causing factors, be it limestone-source water or goiter-causing foods.

When people, especially children, move from a non-goitrous area to a goitrous one, a significant number will develop goiter, some within 6 months of arrival, and others not for 3 or 4 years.[5,6] We saw in

Chapter 4 that goiter development was slow even in a goitrous location such as Pithoragarh. It could take a few years before it develops in a few individuals, while in a few others it may develop rapidly. This varies from individual to individual. The recovery from thyroid disease could similarly vary from individual to individual. The time taken for cure could be short in a few individuals and long in other individuals.

It must be noted that permanent impairment of thyroidal function is an exception; recovery of the gland to the normal state of activity is the rule.[7] It is extraordinary, as American thyroid researcher, David Marine pointed out, that the thyroid can be restored to a comparatively normal functional state even after extreme dysfunction. But the recovery is dependent on the duration of the abnormal process, on the degree of cell death and scarring/injury/damage that may have occurred, on the age of the patient, and state of general nutrition. The thyroid glands of well-nourished children, for example, will recover more quickly and more completely than those of ill-nourished children. In adults in whom the processes of atrophy (degeneration) had already set in, the thyroid is very liable to be impaired permanently by attacks of infectious disease.

Adequate Nutrition in Demanding Life-Stages

We have seen that goiter or thyroid enlargement is most liable to occur during puberty, pregnancy, and lactation. Each of these life-stages puts additional demands on the thyroid gland. Currently, it is common to run thyroid tests during pregnancy and prescribe synthetic thyroid hormone if the diagnostic test values are out of normal range. But people in the past did not have these diagnostic tests or hormone medication, what did they do during pregnancy?

Cultures world over relied on providing good nutrition to pregnant women. In my ancestral village, I once asked a grocery store owner if he had old rice. He asked me if someone was pregnant. Old rice or rice of over a year or more is generally known to be more nutritious than rice that had been harvest recently. Pregnant women were given old rice, as it was more nutritious. Once I attended an agriculture conference in Hyderabad, India. The person sitting next to me was an agriculture scientist of Indian origin who worked for Monsanto in the United States. Monsanto was an American agrichemical company known for their genetically modified seeds. Monsanto was acquired by Bayer, a German company, in 2018. This agriculture scientist told me that his father was a farmer. His father would store paddy (rice with husk) for two years before it was used for home consumption. The long storage period probably reduces the antinutrients and makes the nutrients in rice more available.

Yet another time, I asked a farmer if he had country-chicken eggs. The farmer asked me if I needed them for someone pregnant. Country-chicken eggs are more nutritious than normal poultry-farm chicken eggs. In the past, country-chicken eggs were given to pregnant women as part of a nutritious diet. Both these examples show that local cultures relied on nutritious food to meet the additional demands put on the body during pregnancy. Probably, they also did the same during the other demanding life stages, puberty, and lactation. As the thyroid gland is most liable to be deranged in each of these life stages, it is important to rely on nutritious food during these life-stages, especially among people susceptible to goiter and hypothyroidism in areas supplied by hard water or limestone-source water. Good nutrition is a preventive medicine against thyroid disease in these life-stages.

References

1. Clements FW. Health significance of endemic goitre and related conditions. In: *Endemic Goitre.* Monograph Series No. 44. Geneva: World Health Organization; 1960:13.
2. Inglis J. *Treatise on English Bronchocele: With a Few Remarks on the Use of Iodine and Its Compounds.* London: Longman, Orme, Brown, Green, and Longmans; 1838:10.
3. Kelly FC, Snedden WW. Prevalence and geographical distribution of endemic goitre. In: *Endemic Goitre.* Monograph Series No. 44. Geneva: World Health Organization; 1960:178.

4. McClelland J. An inquiry into the nature and causes of goitre. In: *Some Inquiries in the Province of Kemaon, Relative to Geology and Other Branches of Natural Science.* Calcutta: Thacker & Co. & Cantor & Co.; 1835:315.

5. Major RH. A history of medicine. Springfield. 1954. In: Clements FW, Health Significance of Endemic Goitre and Related Conditions. *Endemic Goitre.* Monograph Series No. 44. Geneva: World Health Organization; 1960:.236.

6. Parra H. *Amer] Public Health.* 1948;38:820. In: Clements FW, Health Significance of Endemic Goitre and Related Conditions. *Endemic Goitre.* Monograph Series No. 44. Geneva: World Health Organization; 1960:236.

7. McCarrison R. *The Thyroid Gland in Health and Disease.* New York: William Wood & Company. 1917:50.

Chapter 11

A Few Helpful Medicines

i. Sunlight

Cretins instinctively sought sunlight.[1] In the 1800s, many observers in the Alps mountains noted that cretins spent their day looking at the sun. Sunlight was somehow helping them. The cretins were probably medicating themselves with sunlight.

Jaundice was noted as a common symptom in newborn cretins in New York in the 1890s.[2] The age-old treatment practiced by midwives in India for newborn jaundice was to expose the babies to sunlight. The exposure to sunlight resolved the jaundice symptoms.

Rickets is a disease in which the bones are deformed in children. In cretinism too, most bones are deformed. In hypothyroidism, the bones are brittle and there are joint pains. In the past, sunlight was used as a medicine in the treatment of rickets in the United Kingdom. British doctors would send children with rickets to spend their day in the open, exposed to sunlight. This resolved rickets symptoms.

Rickets and goiter shared the same geography. Where cretinism prevailed, rickets was found, and where neither goiter nor cretinism was present, rickets was rarely seen.[3] Therefore, the cause of both these diseases is likely the same, i.e., limestone-source water. If sunlight helps in rickets, it has to be helpful in thyroid disease too.

The medicinal role of sunlight in cretinism, newborn jaundice in cretins, and rickets shows that sunlight could act as a medicine in hypothyroidism, as cretinism is nothing but a severe form of thyroid disease.

For a moment, let us step back and look at the role of sunlight in overall health before we look at the role of sunlight in thyroid health. You may have noticed that my name is Suresh. I was named after Suryanarayana, my grandfather (my father's father). *Surya* in my grandfather's name literally means "the Sun" and *Narayana* means "God." My grandfather was named after the Sun God about 100 years ago. His name was a common name during his time. About 2,000 years ago, in the Roman Empire, there was a saying, "where the Sun enters, disease does not enter." You may have never heard of the place where I come from in India. But what is common between such a remote place and the mighty Roman Empire is the importance given to the Sun. The Sun was worshipped across cultures.

People built temples for the Sun God. One of the oldest Sun temples in India was built 1,300 years ago, at Arasavalli, Srikakulam, about 100 kilometers from where I stay on the East coast of India. The largest Sun temple in India was built about 800 years ago in the year 1250, at Konark, on the East coast of India. Similarly, there were Sun temples built in China and Egypt 500 to 2,000 years ago. Any modern man with a scientific bent of mind would have called such practices of praying to the Sun, building temples for the Sun, and naming children after the Sun as a superstition and blind faith. What our forefathers were doing for all these thousands of years may appear irrational. But they must have realized the importance of Sun in the growth of their crops, their livestock, and their own lives.

Vitamin D was discovered only about 100 years ago. In 1925 it was found that sunlight produced Vitamin D in human body. Initially, Vitamin D was considered important for bone health. Later, Vitamin D, and thus sunlight, was proved to be important for the immune system. Anything that is important for the immune system would be beneficial for overall health.

Science was thousands of years late in telling us what our forefathers knew through personal experience and observation. They may not have called it vitamin D. This shows that we may not always be able to explain everything with present-day science. Sometimes we may have to trust personal experience, observation, and traditional practice. It doesn't mean we are being unscientific. In fact, it may mean we are being scientific by accepting that we may not know everything yet. It is just like the local people believed thousands of years ago that water from certain sources caused goiter/thyroid disease.

Sunlight and Endocrine System

Sunlight stimulates the endocrine system.[4] Sunlight directly affects three glands located in the brain—the pituitary gland, the hypothalamus, and the pineal gland. Through these three glands, sunlight stimulates all other endocrine glands.

The photosensitive cells in the retina connect the eyes to the pituitary gland, which is sometimes called *the master gland*, because it controls the functions of all other endocrine glands, such as the thyroid gland and the adrenal gland.

The photosensitive cells in the retina also transmit sunlight to the hypothalamus. The hypothalamus regulates the circadian rhythm, an internal biological clock that helps to anticipate and adapt to the regular rhythm of the day.[5] Our biological rhythm is synchronized with sunlight. The hypothalamus receives nerve messages from the brain, which in turn receives nerve messages from all over the body. The hypothalamus translates these nerve messages into chemical messages and relays them to the pituitary gland.[6] The pituitary gland receives these messages and sends chemical messages to the other endocrine organs. Thus, one of the most important functions of the hypothalamus is to link the nervous system to the endocrine system via the pituitary gland. In addition, the hypothalamus acts like a thermostat: it ensures consistent maintenance of internal body functions by monitoring temperature, blood pressure, water balance, reproductive behaviors, appetite, and mood.[8] All these functions are disrupted in thyroid disease. Thus, the hypothalamus has functions that are related to thyroid disease. As sunlight affects the hypothalamus, it has a role in thyroid function.

The pineal gland has light-sensitive cells. Darkness stimulates the pineal gland to produce a hormone called melatonin. Light, whether sunlight or artificial light, impedes secretion of melatonin. Melatonin secretion gradually starts to increase from 7 p.m. in the evening, reaches a peak production between 3am and 5 am in the night, and gradually declines up to 10 a.m. Negligible amounts of melatonin are produced during the day. At 9 pm, the presence of melatonin hormone can be measured in the blood or saliva.[7] Melatonin is involved in maintaining circadian rhythm. We sleep for 8 hours, once in 24 hours; we do not sleep for 16 hours, once in 48 hours. Although the sleep time is the same in both these scenarios, the body rhythm is tuned to the sun's cycle of 24 hours. Similarly, the human body tunes itself to the tidal, seasonal, and annual rhythms of the environment through sunlight, hypothalamus, and pineal gland. Melatonin also affects the timing of significant hormonal changes (such as *when* puberty starts).[8] The thyroid gland plays a key role during puberty, and sunlight, through melatonin, affects puberty.

Yet another way sunlight and thyroid gland are inextricably linked is through calcitonin. Calcitonin is a hormone secreted by the thyroid gland and is involved in maintaining calcium levels in the body. We also know that sunlight plays an important role in calcium metabolism; it is required to absorb calcium from food in the intestine.

In a way, sunlight is like the conductor of the symphony of hormones in the body. Hormones in turn affect physiological functions such as digestion, growth, metabolism, reproduction, and excretion.

Artificial Light

Just as natural sunlight acts as a medicine in thyroid disease and plays a role in the functioning of the endocrine system, artificial light in our homes and offices disrupts the normal functioning of the endocrine system. Below is an example that shows how artificial light disrupts hormones.

In our ancestral village in India, next to a parcel of agriculture land we own is a broiler-chicken farm. About 15,000 broiler-chickens are grown for meat in the 2-acre farm. Broiler-chicken is a cross-bred genetic-variety, designed for fast growth in weight.

After sunset, the chicken-farm owner switches on incandescent light bulbs in the huts where the chicken are grown. He keeps the lights on throughout the night. He switches them off after sunrise. The chicken in this farm grow to a weight of about 2 kg (kilograms) in 1.5 months. A native country-chicken-breed growing in the open in our village typically attains the same weight in 6–8 months. The light from incandescent bulbs throughout the night for 1.5 months makes the chicken eat more food, and it is one of the reasons for the abnormal and fast growth in weight of the broiler chicken in comparison with the country chicken. The other reasons are selective breeding for fast growth (i.e., breeds that grow fast) and the excess food (especially soy) that broiler chicken get relative to country chicken. The average weight of broiler chickens at 56 days in the United States was approximately 1 kg in 1957, 2 kg in 1978, and 4 kg in 2005.[9]

The poultry industry also uses artificial light to increase egg production. Artificial lights are used during the winter to lengthen daylight hours and thus to increase egg production. We may note how artificial light leads to increased egg production, which is actually a sexual activity.

In both the above examples, *growth* and *sexual activity* were manipulated using artificial light. In other words, the growth hormones and sexual hormones could be manipulated by artificial light.

We are doing to ourselves what we are doing to the broiler-chicken in the poultry farm. We continuously spend our life under artificial light. Lights in our homes, offices, shops, computers, televisions, and mobile phones focus artificial light on our eyes through day and night. The master glands in the brain, pituitary gland, pineal gland, and hypothalamus are evolutionarily not accustomed to artificial light, especially at night, when they expect darkness.

The pineal gland, for example, expects darkness in the late evening/night to secrete melatonin hormone. However, use of artificial light after sunset, leads to reduced secretion of melatonin. Reduced melatonin disrupts the circadian rhythm of the body and the associated physiological functions. As melatonin is involved in puberty, we can only imagine the constant exposure to artificial light has on sexual development during puberty, the life-stage in which the thyroid gland is greatly involved.

Let us assume that after sunset our thyroid gland normally operates at half its potential in comparison with its operating potential during the day. But because of the artificial light in the evening, the master gland may instruct the thyroid gland to operate at its full potential. All other glands will have to adjust their functioning accordingly. As a result, the biological functions of metabolism, growth, reproduction, digestion, and excretion are disrupted. These changes may not happen if we expose ourselves to artificial light for a few hours or days. But prolonged exposure to artificial light as in the case of the poultry-chicken may eventually result in disease.

The trouble is not just the increase in functioning of the thyroid gland after sunset, it is difficult to estimate the quality of thyroid hormone secretion under artificial lights. For example, LED lights that are commonly used today for lighting, television, mobiles, and computers, flicker on and off continuously. The flicker is so fast that we do not normally notice the flicker. But the brain registers the flicker. Similarly, the radio frequency energy from fluorescent tube lights has been recorded in EEG readings of human brain waves.[4(p228)] We can only speculate the impact of the constant on–off flicker signals from LED lights on our brain and glands. Does the flicker result in start and stop instructions continuously to the thyroid gland too? What impact does it have on the functioning of all other glands and their respective secretions?

There is another problem with artificial lights. They do not display the full spectrum of light as does sunlight. For example, sunlight has other components in it—ultraviolet (UV) rays and infrared waves. These rays and waves are not visible to the human eye. Ultraviolet is shorter in wavelength than visible light, and infrared is longer in wavelength than visible light. Generally, ultraviolet rays are considered harmful. But they are also useful. The commonly used window glass obstructs ultraviolet rays. Flowers of plants grown in glass greenhouses do not bloom well, while plants grown in plastic greenhouses that allow UV rays bloom well.[4(p10)] Similarly, in experiments, apples on apple trees shielded in glass enclosures do not ripen due to obstruction of UV rays.[4(p31)] These examples show the complex ways in which sunlight affects life. Artificial lights (LED lights, fluorescent tube lights, and incandescent bulbs) usually do not display ultraviolet rays. Hence, they do not display full the spectrum light as does sunlight.

Artificial lights usually display light in a dominant color. The dominant color emitted by incandescent bulbs is in the spectrum of red/orange/pink/yellow. It does not have blue light. What happens when we are continuously exposed to one dominant color of light? We have seen how incandescent bulbs affect growth and egg production (reproductive function) of chickens in a poultry farm.

Now, let's consider one particular color—pink light—and see how it affects the endocrine system. All over the world, pink is the favorite color of women. It may not be purely for fashion reasons that women like pink. There may be a strong biological reason why women like pink color. The following were the observations and experiments conducted by John Ott, an American researcher, who made significant contributions to our understanding of the impact of light on plants, animals, and man.[4] His observations and experiments show the impact of exclusive exposure to pink light on fertility, mental health, and behavior.

Pink light affects fertility in animals. In an experiment, 8 pairs of mice were kept in a room where they received normal daylight filtered through ordinary window glass, 30 pairs of mice were kept in a dark room lit only by daylight white-fluorescent tubes, and 30 pairs of test mice were kept in another dark room lit only by pink-fluorescent tubes.[4(p69)]

The offspring of mice under normal daylight filtered through ordinary window glass and the offspring of mice under the white fluorescent light consisted of 6–15 offspring, which was the normal number for this particular type of mice. The offspring of mice under pink-fluorescent light consisted of only 1 or 2 offspring. That is, pink light had drastically reduced the number of offspring. It is surprising that a specific color of light can affect fertility so drastically. The pink light had an effect on the sexual hormones, and the effect was seen in the reduced number of offspring.

Minks are small animals weighing about 600 grams to 1 kilogram. They are farm-bred in the United States and Europe for their fur for use in clothing. Minks are by nature quite fierce. When the minks were exposed to natural daylight through a deep pink glass, they became very aggressive.[4(p124-125)] When some of the minks were placed behind deep blue plastic, they became friendly/docile. Normally fierce animals becoming docile is an unnatural thing. Thus, we may note how different colors of light affect the *behavior* of animals.

In the same experiment, it was found that all the male minks behind the deep blue plastic were found to be "working males," i.e., they could mate and cause pregnancy in females, while 90% of males behind the pink glass were found to be "nonworking". Deep blue color affected *behavior* while pink color affected *fertility*.

Similar observations have been made in humans. When a baseball player's glasses in the Kansas City Royals Baseball Academy were changed from pink-tinted to a medium gray, per recommendation of John Ott, the player changed from a hyperaggressive and helmet-throwing player to a very relaxed, confident person.[4(126-127)] There was a great deal of improvement in performance. Another player who had mysteriously retrograded in performance for no evident reason, had regained his usual good performance after the removal of psychedelic-type red lighting from his dormitory room.

John Ott on a trip to Florida was told by a radio station manager about an experience at their station.[4(123)] The staff at the radio station replaced the regular white fluorescent tubes with deep pink color tubes in the studios and control rooms. About two months later, the radio station began to have personnel problems. Announcers began to perform poorly on the air. Everyone became irritable, were consistently at odds with management decisions, and were generally difficult to control. Two resignations were received from employers without any known reasons. Then, one morning, one of the men said, "If those pink bulbs aren't removed, I will go out of my mind." The same day the pink tubes were removed and replaced with white tubes. Within a week, as if by miracle, tempers ceased to flare, congeniality and a spirit of working together began to redevelop, and the resignations were withdrawn. The work improved, with mistakes at a minimum.

The above observations of John Ott show that artificial color light disrupts reproductive function and behavior in animals and human beings. The way light disrupts these functions is through glands and hormones.

Any treatment for thyroid disease should include adequate exposure to sunlight during the day and no exposure to artificial lights both during the day and at night. Just as we eat food every day, we must be exposed to sunlight every day. It would be naïve to think that a supplement like vitamin D could replace sunlight.

ii. Ayurveda

Ayurveda is an ancient Indian medical system, which is about 2,000 years old. Ayurveda recommends milk, barley, old rice, green gram/lentil, chickpeas, sugarcane juice, and cucumber in the treatment of thyroid disease.[10] Ayurveda also recommends avoiding foods that are sour and heavy, as they can aggravate thyroid disease.[10]

How does milk help in thyroid disease?

Milk likely balances lactic acid and lactate produced in the body during the normal course of metabolism. Lactic acid is an organic acid, and lactate is its conjugate base. Lactate plays a role in maintaining blood plasma pH, which is dependent on strong ion difference.

Strong ion difference may be defined as below.[11]

Strong Ion Difference = [Sodium (Na^+) + Potassium (K^+) + Calcium (Ca^{2+}) + Magnesium (Mg^{2+}) + Hydrogen (H^+)] – [Chloride (Cl^-) + Lactate + Urate]

We may note lactate in the above definition. As lactate changes, strong ion difference changes, and as strong ion difference changes, the pH value changes. Lactate, thus, plays a role in maintenance of plasma pH. And thyroid disease symptoms are caused by changes in plasma pH value.

Lactate is continuously produced in our body during metabolism and exercise.[12] During intense exercise such as sprinting, when the rate of demand for energy is high, glucose is broken down and oxidized to pyruvate, and lactate is then produced from the pyruvate faster than the body can process it, causing lactate concentrations to rise.[13]

Another source of lactic acid/lactate is milk. Shortly after milk is taken from the cow, bacteria start turning milk into lactic acid. There may not be much lactic acid initially, but lactic acid keeps increasing shortly after. By the time the milk reaches us, there is some lactic acid in it. Fermented milk products such as yogurt and cottage cheese have more lactic acid in them. Even sourdough bread has lactic acid in it—it is the lactic acid which gives sour taste to sourdough bread. Thus, the lactic acid/lactate formed in our body by drinking milk likely helps in maintaining plasma pH and thus in addressing thyroid disease symptoms.

Lactate is used as an energy source in the nervous system (brain, spinal cord, and nerves). Although glucose is usually assumed to be the main energy source for living tissues, there are reports that indicate that it is lactate, and not glucose, that is preferentially metabolized by neurons in the brain.[14,15] The extracellular fluid immediately surrounding neurons strongly differs in composition from the blood or cerebrospinal fluid, being much richer with lactate.[10] Some evidence suggests that lactate is important at early stages of development for brain metabolism in prenatal and early postnatal subjects, with lactate (at these stages) being in higher concentrations in body liquids and being utilized by the brain preferentially over glucose.[14] Lactate can also serve as an important source of energy for other organs, including the heart and liver. During physical activity, up to 60% of the heart muscle's energy turnover rate derives from lactate oxidation.[16]

From the above discussion, we can see that lactate provides energy for the functioning of the muscle and nervous systems. Therefore, just as calcium plays a role in muscles and nerves, even lactic acid and lactate play an important role in muscles and nerves. In hypothyroidism, both muscle and nerve functions are disrupted. Therefore, milk, by regulating lactic acid/lactate levels in the body, addresses muscle and nervous symptoms in hypothyroidism.

Milk may play another important role in the context of thyroid disease. Milk is the sole food that a newborn baby takes for many months after birth. Milk has all the nutrients to exclusively sustain a newborn baby. When one drinks milk, one gets the same nutrients that a cow provides to its calf. A healthy cow's milk likely has the right combination of various minerals, vitamins, and other nutrients. While it is true that milk is for calf, not man, at least in thyroid disease, milk seems to provide nutrition in an appropriate proportion to sustain human health, especially in people who drink limestone-source water, and thus are deficient in all nutrients, minerals, micronutrients, and trace elements.

In thyroid disease, good quantity and quality of milk may help in alleviating thyroid disease symptoms. As discussed in the chapter on food and thyroid disease, the quality of milk depends on various factors like the breed of cow, feed, soil, season, and so on. One has to choose milk that suits oneself, and the only way to find milk that suits oneself is through trial and error, as there are so many variables that affect milk.

Ayurveda also recommends avoiding sour foods. Sour foods are acidic. For example, tamarind is a sour fruit, which is widely used to make lentil-based stew, a staple in South India. However, tamarind is avoided by some in North India, as it is known to break the blood. Anything that breaks the blood is harmful in thyroid disease. Thyroid disease, as we have seen earlier, is ultimately caused by diseased state of blood.

iii. Guggenbühl's Treatment

We have seen previously that cretinism was most prevalent in certain valleys of Switzerland. Around the year 1845, Dr. Johann Guggenbühl established a hospital, specifically for the treatment and cure of cretinism at Abendberg, near Interlaken, Switzerland.[17] He was successful in bringing about complete cure in a few cases of cretinism. This provides us hope because cure could be brought about in the most extreme form of thyroid disease, i.e., cretinism. It shows that cure/treatment is possible even in milder forms of thyroid disease, i.e., hypothyroidism.

Dr. Guggenbühl made the following changes in the daily life of cretins at the Abendberg hospital to bring about the cure.[18]

1. Water that was not hard was provided to the patients.
2. The hospital was constructed at a height of 4,000 feet above sea level. Cretinism never occurred, or rarely occurred, above this altitude. The air was pure, dry, and unconfined in comparison with the closed valleys where the air was stuck and languid and where many cretins were found. The fresh air acted as a medicine.
3. Exercise in the open air was practiced. In winter, exercise was done in the hall of the hospital. It was noticed that cretins took great pleasure in exercise.
4. Cleanliness, constant washing, and bathing were used in the treatment of cretinism. Hot baths were useful in treatment. Cold baths were found to do more harm than good. The action of the skin was further excited by brushing and friction with aromatic spiritous liquids, which are rubbed into the back and extremities morning and evening.
5. Magnetism and electromagnetism were employed to excite the body.
6. Cretins were easily chilled and almost always had cold hands and feet. On this account, they were warmly clad, usually in wool.

7. The diet was nourishing and abundant. At Abendberg, the patients received milk, rice, meat, nourishing roots (except potatoes), and white bread.
8. The diet roll was the following. Breakfast was goat's milk and white bread. Lunch was milk and rice soup or meat broth, vegetables, veal, beef, mutton (very tender, cut into small pieces). In the afternoon, there was tea of herbs, milk, bread, or fruit. For dinner, it was milk soup, meat broth, or egg soup. The patients always had a large appetite, which was larger in proportion to the degree of their illness. Freshwater as well as milk was given in abundance.

Overall, the progress was slow, often, the steps of improvement were few and far, and patience was required. The process of mental cure was longer, more tedious, and less promising than the physical cure. Dr. Guggenbühl desired that the patient be at the establishment not less than 3 years to do justice to his treatment, though some may have required 5 or 6 years of treatment. So, successful was his treatment that out of the patients he had, a third left completely cured.

iv. Breathing Exercises

Limestone source water disturbs the balance of carbon dioxide and bicarbonate in the body. Thus, the balance between oxygen and carbon dioxide is disturbed.

Breathing exercises improve lung capacity and get more oxygen into the body. This helps in balancing the oxygen and carbon dioxide levels in the body. In India, ancient sages noticed that animals with a slow breath rate (such as pythons, elephants, and tortoises) had a long-life span, whereas those with a fast-breathing rate (such as birds, dogs, and rabbits) lived only a few years.[19] From this observation, they realized the importance of slow breathing for increasing the human life span. Such observations were codified in *Pranayama*, which means breath control. Pranayama breathing exercises may also help in thyroid disease by bringing oxygen and carbon dioxide balance. One may find many pranayama exercises on YouTube.

Living in closed rooms, ill-ventilated homes, and offices reduces the overall availability of oxygen. The successful experience of Dr. Guggenbühl in providing pure and unconfined air in treatment of cretinism shows that adequate fresh air will be helpful in addressing hypothyroidism symptoms.

v. Earthing/Grounding

In the section on electrolytes, we noted that electrolytes (e.g., sodium, potassium, calcium) have electric charge associated with them. A few electrolytes have positive charge, and a few have negative charge. In thyroid disease, there is an imbalance in the electrolytes in extracellular and intracellular fluids. Consequently, there is a disturbance in the electric charge in the body. But per the principle of electroneutrality, the positive charged ions and negative charged ions should be equal. In blood plasma, electroneutrality is always maintained by the body.

Earth is an electromagnet. An electromagnet is a type of magnet in which the magnetic field is produced by electric current. The Earth's magnetic field is a result of the movement of liquid iron in the Earth's crust. As the liquid iron moves, it generates electric currents, which create a magnetic field.[20] The continual movement of liquid iron through this magnetic field creates stronger electrical currents and thus stronger magnetic fields.

Even sunlight is an electromagnet. We have discussed at length at how important sunlight is in helping resolve thyroid disease symptoms. It is the electromagnetic property of sunlight that helps in thyroid disease; similarly, the electromagnetic property of the Earth can be helpful in thyroid disease.

Earthing or grounding is walking on earth barefoot. Walking barefoot on the earth helps one connect with the magnetic balance of the earth. As walking barefoot is how we have evolved over millennia, walking barefoot brings an electrical balance in the body through the magnetic balance of the earth. This is like how electromagnetic property of sunlight brings chemical balance in the human body. The electromagnetic light energy of the sun is converted into chemical energy in the body. Similarly, the electromagnetic energy of the earth brings electrical and chemical balance in the body.

vi. Food

As discussed in the chapter on food and thyroid disease, adequate quantity and quality nutrition offers protection against thyroid disease. Hence, when one is already suffering from thyroid disease, one may focus on getting good nutrition to address thyroid disease symptoms. At the same time, one may avoid overly processed grains and common goiter-causing foods such as cassava, millets, soyabean, peanuts, and vegetables such as cauliflower, cabbage, kale, etc. One must observe how one feels after eating a particular food and then decide for oneself whether it agrees with them or not.

There is no magic pill for thyroid disease, and there will never be. When even normal thyroid gland function fluctuates with season, life-stage, and place of residence, one cannot expect to have a standard pill that works in all seasons, in all life-stages, and in all places of residence. One must change one's food and lifestyle habits in accordance with the season, life-stage, and place of residence.

Emma Morano was an Italian supercentenarian who lived to the age of 117. She was the oldest living person when she died in 2017. When she was a child, she lived in Ossola, Italy. Ossola is located at the foothills of the Alps Mountain range. It is surrounded by Swiss and Italian Alps on the western side, the eastern side, and the northern side.[21] The western side Alps are in Canton of Valais (in Switzerland), and in Piedmont and the Asota valley (in Italy). Canton of Valais, as we have seen in the chapter on geographical distribution of goiter and cretinism, was the most severely affected endemic region of Switzerland. One in twenty-five inhabitants of the canton of Valais were cretins. Similarly, in 1883, in the province of Piedmont, one in every 67 inhabitants were either goitrous or had cretinism. Morano, in her childhood, lived in a such great endemic region. When she was around 18 years of age, she was diagnosed with anemia.[22] This is not a surprise, given what we discussed earlier. Anemia is a common symptom of hypothyroidism. Given the geographical and geological background of where she lived, we may infer that her anemia was likely due to hypothyroidism. The climate of her location—humid and cold winters—was not congenial to her constitution, and so a doctor suggested that she move to the nearby environment of Lake Maggiore.[23] She chose Verbania, a lakeshore town with a milder climate. The doctor also recommended that she eat three eggs and one banana every day. She ate three eggs, two of them raw, and one banana for the next 90 years. She was estimated to have eaten over 100,000 eggs during her lifetime.[24] One reason eggs may help in thyroid disease may be because of the optimal selenium content. T_4 is converted to the active T_3 within cells by selenium-containing enzymes, and thus dietary selenium is essential for T_3 production. Also, eggs optimal levels of fat, protein, and energy. Change of air (probably there was a change of water source too with change of place), three eggs, and one banana was all that the doctor recommended to Morano for her anemia (probably, caused by hypothyroidism). And she went on to live a healthy life till the age of 117.

vii. Naming of Diseases

"A rose called by any other name would smell as sweet." This is what Shakespeare wrote in Romeo and Juliet. The inherent quality of a rose doesn't change if we call it by some other name.

In childhood, my name was Narendra Kumar. My father changed my name to Suresh when my grandfather died, and I was named after my grandfather. I am the same person whether my name is Narendra Kumar or Suresh.

In medicine, however, naming of a disease matters. Depending on the name given to a disease, the medication changes accordingly. If thyroid disease is called an autoimmune disease, then medication to suppress the immune system is given to the patient. If thyroid disease is called hypothyroidism, then synthetic thyroid hormone is given as medicine to the patient.

We have seen that there is a long list of symptoms in hypothyroidism. Any set of symptoms could be selected and given a new name. For example, one set of symptoms in hypothyroidism is related to muscles and rheumatic joint pains, which is commonly called by the name rheumatoid arthritis. When called by this name, the treatment may involve immune-system-suppressing drugs as rheumatoid arthritis is considered to be an autoimmune disease.

Goiter and cretinism were the names used for thyroid disease for a long time. Local people the world over had used local names for these diseases. In the United States and other nonendemic regions, the name "sporadic cretinism" was used instead of "cretinism" for the same symptoms. In 1873, William Gull, a physician at Guy's Hospital, London, first described hypothyroidism in adults as "a cretinoid state supervening in the adult life of a woman."[25] Note that he used the word cretinism to describe hypothyroidism. In 1877, William Ord, London, proposed the name "myxodema" or "mucous oedema," for the adult condition of cretinism-like symptoms.[26] Mucous edema refers to build-up of fluid in the body. Ord likely used this name to refer to the puffy face and bloated body that one normally sees in hypothyroidism.

In 1912, Hakaru Hashimoto, a Japanese doctor, described four symptoms that were later named as Hashimoto thyroiditis. These symptoms were a build-up of white blood cells in thyroid gland (lymphocytic infiltration), eosinophil changes (eosinophils are also a type of white blood cells), reduction in the size of thyroid gland tissues (parenchymal atrophy), and a swollen/damaged thyroid gland (fibrosis). As we have seen throughout this book, blood-related changes are common in thyroid disease, especially those related to white blood cells, lymphocytes, and eosinophils. The other two symptoms that Hashimoto described, reduction in size of thyroid gland tissue and swollen/damaged thyroid gland, occur commonly in thyroid disease. Therefore, based on these four prominent symptoms, the disease was given a new name. The diagnosis for Hashimoto's could only be made by a surgeon on the operation table or when a part of thyroid gland was removed during autopsy, and therefore not many were diagnosed with Hashimoto's in the past. Subsequently, with development of needle biopsy, thyroid tissue could be easily taken without the need for a surgery, and thus more patients were diagnosed with Hashimoto's. In 1950s, it was found that the blood plasma of Hashimoto patients had antibodies against proteins made in the thyroid gland. Hence, the disease was named as an autoimmune disease.

Thus, over the last 150 years, the same disease or set of symptoms was called by different disease names, depending on the symptoms the researcher focused on. Better technical equipment may have enabled us to measure antibodies, but the inherent nature of the disease, i.e., the symptoms that matter to the patient, did not change. Since the treatment changes with the name of the disease, it is important to focus on addressing the cause of the disease, rather than focusing on the name of disease. Addressing the cause will address the symptoms, whatever be the disease name.

References

1. Wells E. *Essay Upon Cretinism and Goiter.* London: John Churchill; 1845:51.
2. Koplik H. Sporadic cretinism and its distinction from forms of idiocy and other diseases. *NY Med J.* Sept 4, 1897.
3. Maffei. *Der Kretinismus in den Norischen Alpen*. Erlangen; 1844:179.
4. Ott JN. *Health and Light.* Indore, India: Banyan Tree; 2012.
5. Press release. The Nobel Prize in physiology or medicine 2017. The Nobel Prize. https://www.nobelprize.org/prizes/medicine/2017/press-release/. Accessed May 18, 2022.
6. Pituitary gland. Endocrine surgery. https://endocrinesurgery.ca/the-endocrine-system/pituitary-gland/. Accessed May 8, 2022.
7. Circadian rhythm. Wikipedia. https://en.wikipedia.org/wiki/Circadian_rhythm. Accessed May 8, 2022.

8. Anatomy of the endocrine system. Stanford Children's. Health. https://www.stanfordchildrens.org/en/topic/default?id=anatomy-of-the-endocrine-system-85-P00401. Accessed May 2, 2022.

9. Zuidhof et al. Growth, efficiency, and yield of commercial boilers from 1957, 1978, and 2005. *Poult Sci.* 2014;93(12):2970-2982. doi: 10.3382/ps.2014-04291. In: How chicken became the rich world's most popular meat. The Economist. https://www.economist.com/international/2019/01/19/how-chicken-became-the-rich-worlds-most-popular-meat. Jan 19, 2019 edition. Accessed May 2, 2022.

10. Niazi AK, Kalra S, Irfan A, Islam A. Thyroidology over the ages. *Indian J Endocrinol Metab.* 2011;15(Suppl 2):S121-S126. doi:10.4103/2230-8210.83347.

11. Catalyst University. What is lactate and lactic acid. YouTube. https://www.youtube.com/watch?v=v-g8gqfs3Xk. Accessed May 28, 2022.

12. Summermatter S, Santos G, Pérez-Schindler J, Handschin C. Skeletal muscle PGC-1α controls whole-body lactate homeostasis through estrogen-related receptor α-dependent activation of LDH B and repression of LDH A. *Proc Natl AcadSci USA*;2013;110(21): 8738–8743. In: Lactic Acid. Wikipedia. https://en.wikipedia.org/wiki/Lactic_acid. Accessed May 28, 2022.

13. Lactic Acid. Wikipedia. https://en.wikipedia.org/wiki/Lactic_acid. Accessed May 28, 2022.

14. Zilberter Y, Zilberter T, Bregestovski P. Neuronal activity in vitro and the in vivo reality: the role of energy homeostasis. *Trends Pharmacol Scie.* 2010;31(9):394–401. doi:10.1016/j.tips.2010.06.005. In: Lactic Acid. Wikipedia. https://en.wikipedia.org/wiki/Lactic_acid. Accessed May 28, 2022.

15. Wyss MT, Jolivet R, Buck A, Magistretti PJ, Weber B. In vivo evidence for lactate as a neuronal energy source. *J Neurosci.* 2011;31(20):7477–7485. doi:10.1523/JNEUROSCI.0415-11.2011.

In: Lactic Acid. Wikipedia. https://en.wikipedia.org/wiki/Lactic_acid. Accessed May 28, 2022.

16. Scott PK, Wolfgang MK, Jacques P. Lactate and acidity in the cancer microenvironment. *Annu Rev Cancer Biol.* 2020:4:141–158. doi:10.1146/annurev-cancerbio-030419-033556. In: Lactic Acid. Wikipedia. https://en.wikipedia.org/wiki/Lactic_acid. Accessed May 28, 2022.
17. Twining W (trans.). In: Guggenbuehl JJ. *Extracts From the First Report of The Institution on The Abendburg, Near Interlachen, Switzerland, for The Cure of Cretins*; 1845.
18. Blackie GS. *Cretins and Cretinism,* A Prize Thesis of University of Edinburgh. Edinburgh: Maclachlan & Stewart and London: Simpkin, Marshall & Co.; 1855.
19. Saraswati SS. *Asana, Pranayama, Mudra, Bandha*. Munger, Bihar: Yoga Publications Trust; 2013:374.
20. Nace T. We Finally know how birds can see earth's magnetic field. Forbes. https://www.forbes.com/sites/trevornace/2018/04/04/we-finally-know-how-birds-can-see-earths-magnetic-field/?sh=7387f78720e1. Accessed May 28, 2022.
21. Ossola. Wikipedia. https://en.wikipedia.org/wiki/Ossola. Accessed May 28,2022.
22. World's oldest person, Emma Morano, dies at age of 117. BBC. https://www.bbc.com/news/world-europe-39610937. Accessed May 28, 2022.
23. Povoledo E. Raw eggs and no husband since 38 keep her young at 115. NYTimes. https://www.nytimes.com/2015/02/15/world/raw-eggs-and-no-husband-since-38-keep-her-young-at-115.html. Accessed May 28, 2022.
24. Povoledo E. Emma Morano, world's oldest person, turns 117. NYTimes. https://www.nytimes.com/2016/11/29/world/europe/emma-morano-worlds-oldest-person-turns-117.html. Accessed May 28, 2022.

25. Gull WW. On a cretinoid state supervening in adult life in women. *Trans Clin Soc Lond.* 1874;7:180–185. In: Slater S. The discovery of thyroid replacement therapy. Part 2: The critical 19th century. *J R Soc Med*. 2011: 104: 59–63. DOI 10.1258/jrsm.2010.10k051.

26. Ord WM. On myxoedema, a term proposed to be applied to an essential condition in the "cretinoid" affection occasionally observed in middle-aged women. *Med-Chir Trans.* 1878;61:57-78. In: Slater S. The discovery of thyroid replacement therapy. Part 2: The critical 19th century. *J R Soc Med*. 2011: 104: 59–63. DOI 10.1258/jrsm.2010.10k051.

Chapter 12

Other Diseases Caused by Limestone-Source Water

Deaf Mutism

Deaf mutism is a defining symptom of cretinism. In almost all countries, deaf mutism was used as the selection criteria for identification of cretins.[1(p399)] In Asia, McCarrison noted that deaf mutism was a constant feature in cretinism; it was present in 87% of cretinism cases.[1(p404)] Table 12.1 presents the census figures for goiter and deaf mutism in the year 1901 at the foothills of the Himalayas in India.[2(p1065)]

Table 12.1 Census figures at the foothills of the Himalayas in India for goiter and deaf mutism in the year 1901

Administrative area	Total number of patients attending dispensaries	Goiter cases per 100 patients	Deaf-mute cases per 10,000 patients
Gonda	20,000	5.6	4.7
Tarabganj	30,000	9.1	9.3
Utraula	6,000	1.0	2.7

We may note that the proportion of goiter cases per 100 patients and the proportion of deaf–mutes per 10,000 was practically identical in the administrative areas. The only exception was in the Utraula dispensary, where the proportions were not identical, as a large number of nongoitrous patients from Nepal, which was across the Indian border, visited the dispensary. Similar correlation between goiter and deaf mutism were observed in other endemic areas in Uttar Pradesh, India. Goiter, cretinism, and deaf mutism occupied the same geographies.

Deaf mutism was frequent in families where other family members had cretinism or where parents had goiter.[2(p1066)] The three diseases tended to occur in the affected families. Healthy parents coming to an area of high endemicity produced children with goiters, cretinism, and deaf mutism. If parents moved to unaffected districts, they seldom produced diseased children.

Similar observations were made in the Gilgit area of the Himalayas, where McCarrison made his original observations on goiter disease. Studies found that in this high endemic area, 2.4% of the population were deaf-mutes.[3] In the township of Bettiah, Bihar, India, where the goiter rate among school children was 100%, all 20 deaf–mute cases studied showed goiter, and half of them showed nodular distortion of the thyroid gland.[3]

Rheumatic Joint Pains

Limestone-source water causes rheumatic pains, especially near the bone joints, knee joints, elbow joints, palm joints, and so on.

In our ancestral village in India, people coming from outside the village often complain of joint and muscle pains after a short stay. The same people report that their joint/muscle pains subside on going back to their previous location. The water in our village is primarily from a limestone source. This observation is very similar to observations at a French boarding school, where students got goiter while at the boarding school and lost it during holidays at their hometowns. This is also similar to the observation that tourists to a French holiday destination got holiday goiter, which subsided when the tourists moved back to their hometowns.

In fact, in any muscle, nerve, or bone-related disorder or disease, we have to suspect the involvement of limestone-source water or hard water. Calcium is involved in the function of muscles, nerves, and bones, and the calcium metabolism is disturbed by limestone-source water/hard water.

Squint, Stammering, Mental Deficiencies

Squint, also known as cross-eye or strabismus, was a common symptom in cretins.[1(p395,397,403,407),4] Squint or cross-eye was present in 20% of cretins.[1(p407)]

In modern medicine, squint is usually considered to be caused by weak eye muscles. Accordingly, surgery of eye muscles is the predominant treatment for squint. However, the connection between squint and cretinism shows that squint is caused by limestone-source water. People with squint also show certain social deficits and neurological symptoms rather than mere eye muscle weakness. This shows the relationship between squint and cretinism and thus with limestone-source water.

Stammering was observed to be a common symptom among cretins.[5] Stammering is likely caused by neurological deficits just like squint is.

Impaired mental function is a key symptom in cretinism. Cognitive and intellectual abilities in cretins are absent. Generally, iodine deficiency is said to be the cause of impaired mental abilities in children. But as we have seen throughout this book, it is excess of lime in water that causes the mental deficiencies observed in cretinism. Therefore, excess of lime, rather than deficiency of iodine, may be the cause of various mental deficiencies in children and adults, which were previously ascribed to iodine deficiency.

Infectious Disease

Our bodies are teeming with trillions of microorganisms—bacteria, viruses, fungi and other such small creatures. Different species of bacteria, viruses, and fungi thrive in different pH environments.

Any disturbance of the pH balance in our body creates a conducive environment for certain infectious bacteria and viruses. These infectious bacteria, viruses, and fungi may have a detrimental effect on the thyroid gland and other glands.

In the chapter on Lohaghat and Pithoragarh, we saw that all types of diseases were higher in Pithoragarh, the area of limestone-source water, than in Lohaghat, the area of clay-slate water. The diseases of the intestine were particularly higher in Pithoragarh. The number of dysentery cases was 10 times more in Pithoragarh than in Lohaghat. Dysentery is an infection of the intestines that causes diarrhea. Dysentery is caused by bacteria (shigellosis) or an ameba. Therefore, limestone-source water was eventually leading to infection.

Similar observations were made in London and Scotland. In 1850, in the Report of the London Board of Health on water supply, it was remarked that "since supply of soft water to London, urinary complaints and dyspeptic (indigestion) complaints were less frequent, continued fevers were more seldom and less severe."[6] These fevers included typhoid, typhus, and relapsing fevers, all infection-related fevers.

In Paisley, Scotland, Dr. Paton observed that since the introduction of soft water into that town, which formerly depended on limestone wells, disorders related to water were very rare, while formerly they were very numerous.[6] He also noticed that in the two cholera epidemics, the families using well-water were far more severely afflicted than those using the city water supply, which was soft. Cholera broke out in a suburb, built high and dry on a limestone ridge, the air pure and bracing, drainage excellent, but the water mostly derived from wells sunk in limestone rock. Few persons here escaped cholera, except a few families who had no well water, and therefore had to depend on the city water supply.

After the epidemic at Paisley subsided, it was found that there were 848 cases of cholera. It was estimated that 10% of the population of the town used well-water, and 90% of the population used the city water supply. Of the 10% population that used well-water from a limestone ridge, 502 people got cholera. Of the other 90% population that used the city water supply, 346 people got cholera. Based on the proportion of population, the 10% should have had only 39 cases of cholera instead of 502. This huge difference in excess cholera cases among the 10% population was apparently from using hard water from limestone-water source.

The above discussion shows that limestone-source water/hard water also causes infectious diseases.

Other diseases caused by acid-base imbalance

Most diseases, either caused by an infection or a nutrient deficiency or some genetic disorder, ultimately get reflected in the blood. That is why, when one falls sick, the health of blood is checked by diagnostic tests such as red blood cell count, white blood cell count, the relative concentration of different types of white blood cells, hemoglobin content, the size of blood cells, and platelet count.

Similarly, many diseases should get ultimately reflected in the acid-base level of blood plasma i.e., in the pH value of plasma. The normal plasma is slightly alkaline with a pH of 7.4, with the normal range between 7.35 and 7.45. In any disease, the plasma may be more alkaline than normal or more acidic than normal.

In hypothyroidism disease, the plasma is more alkaline than normal. In hyperthyroidism, the plasma is more acidic than normal. Hyperthyroidism shares many symptoms with diabetes and tuberculosis. A significant loss in body weight, loss of muscle, excessive urination, and excessive sweating are common to all the three diseases—hyperthyroidism, diabetes, and tuberculosis. Often, hyperthyroidism disease is confused with diabetes and tuberculosis because of the common symptoms. Since hyperthyroidism is caused by excess acidic nature of plasma (i.e., low pH), are diabetes and tuberculosis also because of excess acidic nature of plasma?

Diabetes is commonly considered to be caused by insufficient insulin hormone produced by the pancreas or inability of cells in the body to respond to the insulin produced. Let us explore a different probable cause.

The stomach acid has a pH value of 2 i.e., it is 100,000 times more acidic than pure water. When the digested food from the stomach enters the duodenum (the starting 10-15 inches of the small intestine), the food is still highly acidic. The high acidity of chyme (food plus stomach acid) is neutralized in the duodenum by the pancreatic juice released by the pancreas. About 1.5-2 liters of pancreatic juice is secreted each day. Pancreatic juice is alkaline in nature i.e., opposite of acidic nature of stomach acid. The pancreatic juice has water, digestive enzymes, and high concentration of sodium bicarbonate. Sodium Bicarbonate is a base. It neutralizes the highly acidic chyme.

Just as chloride ions are used to make stomach acid, sodium ions are used by pancreatic cells to make pancreatic juice. In order to make the pancreatic juice, sodium ions are removed by pancreatic cells from the blood plasma. As sodium ions are removed from the plasma, the strong ion difference of plasma, i.e., the difference between the concentration of sodium ions and chloride ions, $[Na^+] - [Cl^-]$, is reduced. A reduced strong ion difference means reduced plasma pH i.e., plasma becomes more acidic than normal. Thus, the normal digestion process makes the plasma more acidic than normal as sodium ions are used up in neutralizing the acidic chyme.

When one regularly consumes acidic foods (e.g., alcohol), the pancreas is overburdened to make more alkaline pancreatic juice to neutralize the excess acid. The overburdened pancreas may work at a sub-optimal level, including, producing a decreased amount of insulin hormone.

A vicious cycle may set in by regular consumption of acidic foods. More sodium ions have to be removed from plasma to make more of the alkaline pancreatic juice. As more sodium ions are continuously removed from plasma, plasma will continuously remain more acidic than normal. Eventually, the pancreas may not be able to neutralize the acid coming from stomach in the form of chyme. The overall function of pancreas suffers. The pancreas may not be able to produce enough insulin hormone. This vicious cycle may take a long time to set in, perhaps, the reason why the onset of diabetes is usually in late age.

When one consumes protein-rich food, nitrogen-rich food or food grown with excess nitrogenous fertilizer, it generates excess ammonia (i.e., acid ions) in the body which has to be cleared by the kidneys. When the kidneys are unable to clear the excess acid ions, excess acid builds up in the plasma i.e., the plasma pH becomes lower than normal. The significant increase in diabetes incidence is a recent phenomenon, especially, diabetes incidence has increased significantly in the last 50 years or so. The increase in diabetes incidence coincides with increase in protein consumption as societies became more wealthy, increase in consumption of foods grown with excess nitrogenous fertilizers, and increase in consumption of acidic food (e.g., highly processed grains).

This hypothesis that acidic nature of plasma causes diabetes is also supported by the fact that people with hypothyroidism do not usually contract diabetes. The reason could be that hypothyroidism is caused by excess alkaline nature of plasma, so there is not much possibility of someone simultaneously suffering from excess acidic plasma. There may be few exceptions to this general rule.

In metabolism, thyroid hormones work on catabolism (breakdown of large molecules into smaller ones) and pancreas' hormone insulin works on anabolism (building complex molecules from simpler ones). Thus, thyroid hormones and insulin hormones work on the opposite processes in metabolism. This shows that the cause of thyroid disease (hypothyroidism) is likely to be the opposite of the cause of pancreas disease (diabetes). We have established conclusively through this book that high pH causes hypothyroidism, therefore, low pH (i.e., acidic plasma) could be the cause of diabetes.

There is significant emaciation (loss of body weight), excess urination, and excess sweating in diabetes, hyperthyroidism, and tuberculosis. These symptoms show that body is throwing out fluid from the body in excess. The reason could be that the body is trying to achieve balance between fluid-balance and acid-base balance. These symptoms in diabetes are opposite of the symptoms that we see in hypothyroidism, fluid build-up and weight gain. This observation also shows that the cause of diabetes could be the opposite of the cause of hypothyroidism.

Diabetes and high blood-pressure often occur together in the same person. It is said that they are like sisters, where one goes, the other follows. Then, is the cause of high blood-pressure too high acidic nature of blood plasma?

The important finding of this book is that it conclusively proves that an environmental factor (water) is the cause of a hormonal disease (thyroid disease). This shows that probably other hormone diseases (e.g., diabetes) could also be caused by environmental factors (e.g., acidic/protein-rich/nitrogenous food).

The cause of thyroid disease has been an unresolved question for at least three thousand years of written history. I hope we made significant progress in our understanding of the cause of thyroid disease through this book.

I will shortly publish a book on hyperthyroidism. I will subsequently publish on diabetes, tuberculosis, and mental illness, the cause of each of these diseases has a basis in acid-base balance. Acid-base balance, in turn, is dependent on electrolyte balance, principle of electrical neutrality, body temperature/season, and the function of various glands, hormones, and organs. Disruption in any one of these may ultimately get reflected in acid-base balance.

References

1. Pharoah P, Delange F, Fierro-Benitez R, Stanbury JB. Endemic cretinism. In: Stanbury JB, Hetzel BS, eds. *Endemic Goiter and Endemic Cretinism, Iodine Nutrition in Health, and Disease.* John Wiley; 1980.

2. Stott H, Bhatia BB, Lal RS, Rai KC. The distribution and cause of goitre in United Provinces. *Indian J. Med. Res.* 1931;18(4): 1059-1085.

3. Grant IS et al. Report UK/HA/10, International biological program: Wellcome Trust Anglo-Pakistan goitre survey, Manchester, England, University of Manchester Physical Laboratory, 1968. In: Kochupillai N, Ramalingaswami V, Stanbury JB. *Endemic Goiter and Endemic Cretinism, Iodine Nutrition in Health, and Disease.* John Wiley; 1980:105.

4. Delange F, Dunn JT, Glinoer D, eds. *Iodine Deficiency in Europe.* NATO ASI Series (Series A: Life Sciences). New York: Plenum Press; 1993:26, Table 1.

5. Blackie GS. *Cretins and Cretinism,* A Prize Thesis of University of Edinburgh. Edinburgh: Maclachlan & Stewart and London: Simpkin, Marshall & Co.; 1855:64.

6. Sizer NB. Our drinking water. *Proc Med Soc County Kings.* March 1882;Vol. II(i):4.

About the Author

I am from Visakhapatnam, a city on the east coast of India in the state of Andhra Pradesh. My ancestral village is about 20 kilometres from the city. The drinking-water source of the village is primarily from limestone rocks and earth. If we look at the history of thyroid disease, the best research on thyroid disease was done by Theodore Koch, John McClelland, Robert McCarrison, and others, in Switzerland or in India, in the limestone districts. Similarly, my research is based on observations in my ancestral village.

I have lived in Visakhapatnam, Mumbai, and Chennai, all seacoast cities. This has helped me to appreciate the importance of coastal weather or salt air on health. I could appreciate the insight from McCarrison's research why thyroid gland is half the size near the seacoast compared to its size inland. The fact that I lived most of my life in seacoast cities also helped me to appreciate Peter Stewart's acid-base chemistry and the importance of strong ions, sodium and chloride, the constituents of common salt and the key players in determination of acid-base balance.

In short, based on my personal experience, observation, and research, I was able to connect McClelland's limestone research, McCarrison's thyroid gland size insights, and Peter Stewart's acid-base chemistry.

My academic background is in commerce and management. I worked for various firms in India. But neither my academic background nor my work experience prepared me to write this book. For the past decade, I had to deal with real estate thugs who tried to grab our ancestral land. While dealing with these thugs, I had to visit my ancestral village often, and in the process made observations on the impact of limestone-source drinking water on health of local people.

Further, my mother shared few insights about her friends who were taking synthetic thyroid hormone medication. Few of them had given up their medication. This caused hyperthyroidism-like symptoms. The comparison of symptoms between hypothyroidism and hyperthyroidism helped me form the hypothesis for the cause of thyroid disease. The hypothesis was subsequently confirmed by Peter Stewart's acid-base chemistry.

Any progress in thyroid disease can be made only by recognizing the flaws in the existing theories of iodine deficiency and autoimmunity. A few years ago, in a thesis on thyroid disease, I read that in endemic goiter regions both iodine and bromine were deficient. Normally, only iodine was supposed to be deficient, not bromine. As I researched the history of iodine in the context of thyroid disease, it became clear that iodine deficiency theory is flawed, and that iodine deficiency and autoimmunity were symptoms rather than the cause of thyroid disease.